It Worked For Me ...

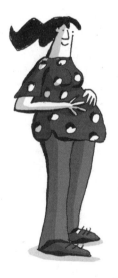

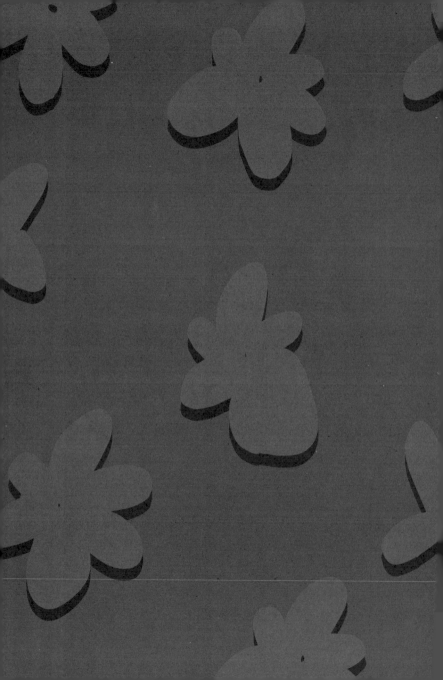

It Worked For Me ...

1001 real-life pregnancy tips

Michelle Kennedy

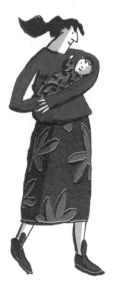

with illustrations by Maddy McClellan

BARRON'S

First edition for the United States,
its territories and possessions, and Canada published in 2004 by
Barron's Educational Series, Inc.
by arrangement with
the Ivy Press Limited

All inquiries should be addressed to:
Barron's Educational Series, Inc.,
250 Wireless Boulevard
Hauppauge, New York 11788
www.barronseduc.com

International Standard Book Number
0-7641-2835-3

Library of Congress Control Number 2003112712

Every effort has been taken to ensure that all information in this book is correct. This book
is not intended to replace consultation with your doctor, surgeon, or other health-care
professional. The author and publisher disclaim any loss, injury, or damage incurred as a
consequence, directly or indirectly, of the use and application of the contents of this book.

This book was conceived,
designed, and produced by
THE IVY PRESS LIMITED
The Old Candlemakers
West Street, Lewes
East Sussex, BN7 2NZ, U.K.

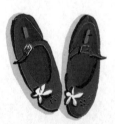

Creative Director *Peter Bridgewater*
Publisher *Sophie Collins*
Editorial Director *Jason Hook*
Design Manager *Tony Seddon*
Senior Project Editor *Rebecca Saraceno*
Editor *Mandy Greenfield*
Designer *Tonwen Jones*
Illustrator *Maddy McClellan*

Printed in China
9 8 7 6 5 4 3 2 1

contents

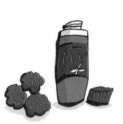

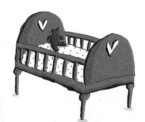

introduction

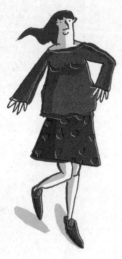

Congratulations! You're pregnant . . . or at least you're thinking about getting pregnant. What an amazing— and sometimes challenging—journey you are embarking upon. Becoming pregnant for the first (or maybe second or third) time is quite an adventure, and one that you will never forget. Don't let anyone fool you into thinking that being pregnant is at all mundane or ordinary, just because women have been doing it for millions of years. It *is* an adventure—and it *is* extraordinary that you are able to bring new life into the world.

From the moment you find out you're pregnant and right up to the moment you finally deliver your baby—even after—you are going to have questions. In fact, if you're at all like me, you will probably question everything: "What is that feeling?" "Is this normal?" "How on earth is a human head supposed to come out of there?!"

Most moms-to-be will have friends and family around them to support them through pregnancy—many of them mothers themselves, who have been through this before. And finding a trustworthy health-care provider—one in whom you feel able to confide— will take you a long way in your journey. A book like this fills another need: you can turn to it when you have odd little questions, like "Why am I peeing all of the time?,"

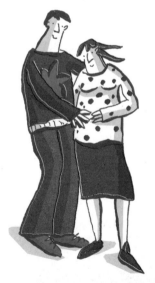

or when you want advice fromsomeone who isn't your mom (or your partner's mom!) and who's actually been there—preferably recently. *It Worked For Me . . .* offers tips that have succeeded for hundreds of moms who have felt exactly the way you do, and who have come through their pregnancies healthily and happily.

A multitude of groups exist out there for new mothers to join. What I find most amazing about women is their ability—within minutes of meeting each other—to pour out all the details of their pregnancies and deliveries. You'll find that complete strangers will walk up to you and tell you whether or not they had an epidural, or whether their heartburn was particularly bad.

It's a crazy group that you're about to join—the land of mothers—but it's a fun one, too. And it will be the most important group you ever belong to, because it will be the most important job you ever have—being a mom. So go ahead: read the tips in this book, learn, and enjoy!

Michelle Kennedy

MICHELLE KENNEDY
2004

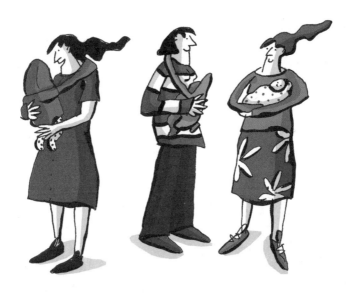

safety tips

You should bear in mind the following safety advice for pregnant women when reading this book:

✋ Although herbal medicine (or phytotherapy) is the oldest form of medicine and is generally considered safe, herbs can have unrecognized effects on pregnancy or labor and may interact with prescribed medicines or have potentially serious consequences for the fetus. Pregnant mothers who wish to consult a medical herbalist should visit one who is registered with a professional body (such as the American Association of Naturopathic Physicians, AANP) and should inform their doctor.

✋ Aromatherapy is the use of the essential oils extracted from various parts of plants. Essential oils are highly concentrated, and when used correctly, most oils are safe; however, certain essential oils carry risks and some are dangerous in pregnancy. Expectant women should therefore consult a trained aromatherapist.

It Worked For Me . . . .

🖐 Homeopathy uses minute doses of substances to boost the body's natural defenses, based on the theory of treating "like with like." Although homeopathic remedies are often thought to be harmless, there are some concerns about their effectiveness and safety. Pregnant women should consult a qualified homeopath.

🖐 Those with a family history of atopy (hypersensitivity, with an inherited tendency to an allergic reaction), or a nut allergy, should consult their health-care provider before eating nuts or peanut butter, because of the risk of an allergy developing in the fetus.

🖐 Pregnant women who follow a well-balanced vegetarian diet that includes milk, eggs (but only well-cooked eggs, not raw or undercooked ones), sufficient calories, and adequate nonmeat sources of iron should be nutritionally satisfied, although vitamin and mineral supplements may be needed; vegans may well need to take supplements of calcium, iron, and vitamin B12.

morning sickness and other ailments

Whoever called it "morning sickness" must have been a man, because he certainly didn't get the all-day, all-the-time, triggered-by-almost-any-food-with-a-smell kind of nausea that I got. And, contrary to popular belief, morning sickness does not end after three months—sometimes not even after four. Most women do finish their bouts of nausea soon after the first trimester, but some unlucky ones don't stop feeling sick until the baby is out.

So, while you're trying out all kinds of experiments to help you guess which sex your baby is (I tried the wedding ring suspended from a chain over my protruding belly; supposedly, if it starts to spin on its own, it's a girl),

morning sickness

you can flip through some hints that many other moms have used to quell that nauseating feeling. And because nausea is not the only ailment you're going to come across during the next nine months (there may be constipation, leg cramps, backache, bladder issues, and lots

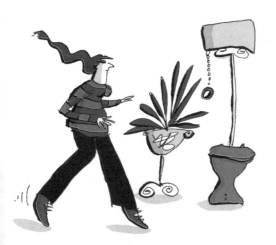

of other fun stuff), we've included tips on those, too. So put away your dread of talking about such subjects and read on.

on the way to work

You may experience feelings of nausea, but not actually vomit, or you may do both. Either way, it's a good idea to plan ahead. One of the first things to consider is how you're going to get safely to and from work. Some women find that eating as soon as they get up makes the ride to work more bearable; deep breathing can also help delay nauseating feelings. If you're feeling too nauseated or dizzy to drive yourself, consider public transportation or car pooling. And try to travel early or late to avoid the rush hour. If you have to drive, make sure you have your car prepared: a bottle of iced water can help, as can driving with the window down or with the cool air directed onto your face. Worst-case scenario: have a couple of plastic grocery bags (without holes!) tucked nearby. And if you are ill, you can freshen up once you arrive at work.

at your desk

You might want to plan the route to the nearest bathroom and keep those plastic grocery bags handy. Even a wastebasket can be useful, and generally there are plenty around. If you're lucky enough to have your own office, you can quietly shut the door. If you work in a cubicle, try to borrow a private, enclosed space or head to the employee lounge or restroom. Cool cloths around your throat and on your forehead may also help the recovery process.

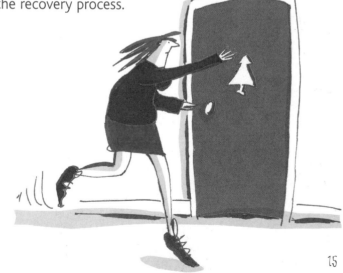

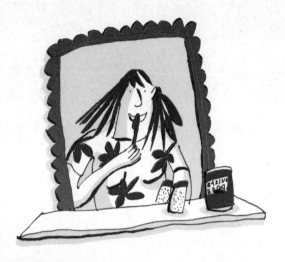

freshen up

To freshen up after a bout of nausea or vomiting, keep a pocket toothbrush or a soft-bristle toothbrush with you. If regular toothpaste is something that is making you feel nauseated, try using children's toothpaste in different flavors. Other speedy breath-freshening techniques are mints or those square sheets of gelatin impregnated with mouthwash, which melt quickly.

enlist some help

You may want to enlist some help from your officemates—for instance, they might be able to cover for you while you step away from your desk. The downside is that, if you wanted to keep the good news a surprise for a while longer, this might make that harder to achieve. If you do ask for help, make sure you place your trust in someone who can keep your secret until you're ready to share it with the world at large.

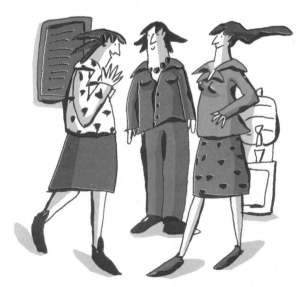

take two

Press two fingers firmly but gently on your belly button, just for a minute, one mom says. This also works for heartburn and is a great tip to use if you're at a restaurant and everything on the menu suddenly looks green. Motion sickness bands are available at boating stores and some pharmacies. These put pressure on wrist points, and are almost guaranteed to cure nausea. And recent studies show that pressure on the pericardium 6 (or P6) point can provide fairly quick relief from nausea. To find this point, place your hand palm up and measure two thumb widths above the most prominent wrist crease; P6 is just above this, in line with your middle finger.

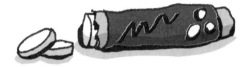

peppermint

Either smelling peppermint in its aromatherapeutic form or sipping the tea can help to curb nausea, and this herb is also known to boost sagging energy levels. For morning sickness, one mom says that the only thing that works for her is scotch mints. "For some reason," she says, "I have a horrible taste in my mouth that makes me feel incredibly ill, and peppermint is the thing that gets rid of that icky taste." Chewing mint gum is a great alternative and can quickly relieve a bout of nausea.

comfort food

Sometimes there is just nothing like a bowl of chicken soup.
That same concoction grandma used to give you, when you ate
too many M&Ms as a girl, has come to the rescue of many a
morning-sick mama! If chicken soup wasn't your thing, then
remember what worked when you were little—you might
find that it not only triggers a soothing feeling, but helps you
get over the mental obstacle that nausea sometimes creates.
One mom swears by salty potato chips, after trying everything
else from saltines to licorice. Have them on hand and be sure to
drink plenty of water to offset the salt. "For two weeks, I could
hardly keep a thing down," another mom said. "I tried just about
everything anyone suggested. Then, on a whim, I went to a
Japanese restaurant and had miso soup. *Surprise!* It settled me
right down, and I was so hungry that I ate a full meal after. The
next morning, it was back to being sick. I went to the Oriental

morning sickness

area of my local grocery and found instant miso soup to test my theory. Now, I have a cup of miso first thing in the morning and am fine for the rest of the day."

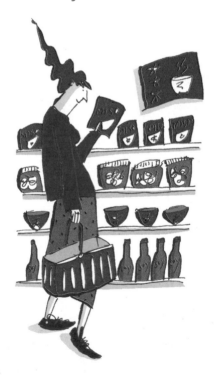

a little tart

Lemons and other citrus fruits have powerful effects. Grating the peel of a lemon (or orange) into a glass of water, or onto a salad, can relieve nausea quickly. If even salad sounds unappealing, try cutting open a lemon and smelling it—one mom swears this helped cure her. You can also try lemon tea or, if you're up for it, sucking on a wedge of lemon. One mom, whose morning sickness lasted all her pregnancy, was helped by a glass of Granny Smith apple juice before she even got out of bed—the tartness helped settle her stomach.

Or try taking a few teaspoons of apple cider vinegar (*not any other kind*) in warm water first thing in the morning.

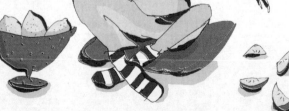

milk shakes

I had morning sickness with all four of my children—a girl and three boys—and those people who told me I would have it only with girls (or boys) were crazy. With my second (my daughter), I wasn't able to eat anything at all and the midwife was getting worried I'd have to go to the hospital for an IV to rehydrate me. Even water made me sick, and I lost 11 lb (5 kg) before gaining any weight (although I did gain it all back—and then some). She told me just to eat anything: at that point, it didn't matter if I ate only chocolate-chip cookies morning, noon, and night! Then I discovered vanilla milk shakes. They were thick enough to quell the acid in my stomach, sweet enough to get me to suck them down, and the vanilla soothed my stomach. I practically lived on them for weeks.

try some tea

A cup of raspberry-leaf tea every day can settle an unnerved
stomach. One herbalist recommends using fresh leaves, if you
can get them (if you have woods near your home, take a walk—
you'll be surprised what you can find, but do please ensure you
know exactly what you're looking for); if not, go to a local co-op
or tea and coffee shop for a pungent dried concoction. Mixing
the tea with cream can also help soothe the stomach and give
it something to work on (instead of you!). Basil leaves and
camomile flowers have been found to soothe nausea, so perhaps
mixing your own combination blend of tea will help.

stick with your cravings

In the beginning, some women are so concerned with eating the "right" things for their baby that they end up throwing them all up! Important though it is to eat well throughout your pregnancy, you may have trouble keeping anything down in the early months, so feel free to listen to your body. If you are craving something (double chocolate whatever, Ben and Jerry's ice cream, a steak), then go eat it! It's better to eat something rather than nothing at this point, and if it makes you feel better, you'll have quelled the queasiness long enough to eat a banana or maybe even a whole salad!

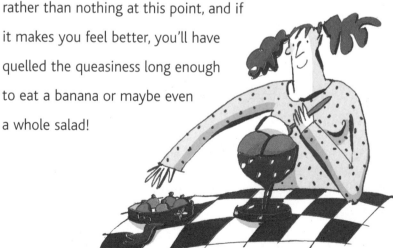

something to stick to your ribs

If you can, eat a peanut-butter sandwich with a warm glass of milk before bed (unless, of course, you have an allergy to nuts or a family history of atopy). This will give your stomach something to work on overnight and ideally, will last you right through until the morning. Keep some bread or crackers by your bed and, if you can, wake yourself up during the night to munch . . . This isn't a great habit to get into for losing weight later on, but it can keep you from running to the bathroom all morning.

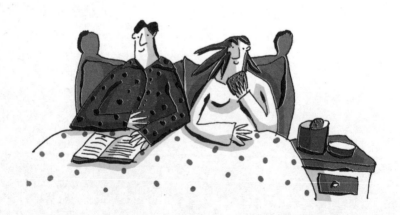

go jump in the lake

One mom swears by swimming to stave off morning sickness. A 30–45-minute swim not only relieves her nausea, but gives her energy for the rest of the day. Joining a local health club with a pool, or even taking an early morning bath, may help. Try to get into a routine whereby you stop at the pool on the way to or from work. Many health clubs also have child-care facilities, if you have a little one at home to worry about. Swimming is not too strenuous and helps to relieve back pain, leg cramps, and other ailments.

toothpaste traumas

Brushing my teeth in early pregnancy was a horror. I have the world's worst gag reflex anyway, and just placing the toothbrush in my mouth sent me to the toilet (of course, this could set up a comical chain of events: throwing up, brushing teeth, and so on and on). If it's the toothpaste itself that is setting you off, try a natural substitute: Tom's of Maine is a soothing natural alternative. One mom told me that resorting to baking soda and salt instead of toothpaste really helped her to get through those first few weeks.

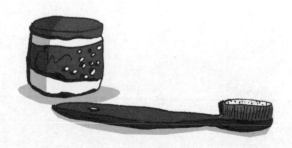

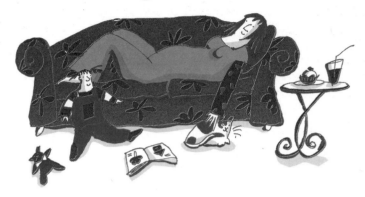

sleep therapy

Sleep your way through morning sickness. Okay, this won't be possible for many people, but if you can, it *does* work. I found that if I didn't move, I was all right. I set myself up on the couch and just lay there—sometimes until noon (I'm not proud of it, but I didn't throw up!). I would bring to the couch everything my little one needed—spare diapers, juice, granola bars—and spent many a morning watching TV, catching a snooze, and reading to my child. This kept the spins to a minimum, and by afternoon I was (mostly) able to make it up to my child by going to the park.

buy premade meals

If food preparation is just too much for you, head to the frozen food section of your local store (frozen foods don't have any smell). There are family-size meals and individual sizes, appetizers and desserts, and most are reasonably priced. And if you can, try to enlist a willing friend or relative (mom!) to bake an extra casserole or two, because this can be a lifesaver in a nauseated moment when there are others to be fed.

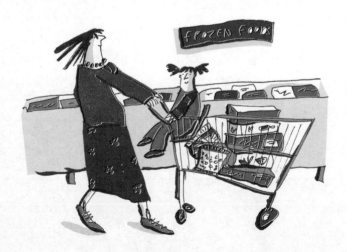

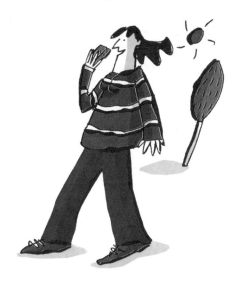

a little bit all day long

Keep food around the house or office. By nibbling a little all day, and having a small meal every two or three hours, you should be able to keep the stomach churning at bay. This strategy also helps you avoid heartburn and other gaseous ailments. And take your time to enjoy a meal: eat slowly and get up from the table slowly—don't rush to do the dishes . . .

homeopathic remedies

These homeopathic preparations may be helpful (for advice on using homeopathy during pregnancy, *see page 11*). Consult your primary health-care provider before using any homeopathic remedy, and alert them immediately if any symptoms change. Homeopathic preparations are available in pharmacies and health-food stores (6C is considered a low-potency remedy):

✋ Ipecacuanha 6: For nausea accompanied by hot or cold, clammy perspiration, and retching; or if you feel better with open air, cool conditions, rest, and keeping still, but worse with eating, excessive heat, damp weather, vomiting, movement, or strong smells.

✋ Colchicum 6C: Good if you have no appetite or feel nauseated by even the thought or smell of food, or feel bloated.

✋ Natrum mur 6C: Worth trying if you belch and can taste what you've eaten, crave salt, and feel thirsty; if you are better for being in the open air, taking rest, going without regular meals, getting peace and quiet, but bad in the late morning, and worse for hot atmospheres, dampness, mental exertion, eating fatty or starchy food, noise, music, touch, or pressure.

Sepia 6C: Use this remedy if you're vomiting, irritable, exhausted, indifferent, chilly or weepy, and have cold clammy periods or hot flashes; if your symptoms are better for eating small amounts, exercise, keeping busy, elevating your legs, and getting fresh air, but bad during the afternoon and worse for the smell of food, fasting, the emotional demands of others, or loss of sleep. For other suggested remedies for nausea, ask your homeopath.

extra zing?

One mom's theory is that you're nauseated because of the excess acid in your tummy. "Food would cure it, but food doesn't even *sound* good when you're that sick. I start out every morning trying to find the one thing that sounds good—or, if not good, then at least not nauseating . . . I eat that as soon as I can, and I'm fine for the rest of the day. Do this early, though. Once I'm in full morning sickness onset, there's no going back." So go with whatever food appeals to you, however unpalatable it may seem to others.

ginger up

Ginger is a natural stomach soother for all kinds of nausea, but you need to take it before you vomit, or it won't stay down. Some women only have to sniff fresh ginger-root to reap the benefits. Making ginger tea—by infusing two teaspoons of grated ginger in a cup of boiling water (sweetened with honey or lemon to taste)—can also help. If you're out of the house and can't brew up, any food item containing ginger should help. Some women swear by stale ginger ale; others prefer the crystallized ginger that is available in cooks' stores. Still other moms use ginger liberally in cooking.

a little aromatherapy

If smell seems to trigger
your nausea, try the
following aromatherapeutic
suggestions (for advice on
using aromatherapy in
pregnancy, *see page 10*):

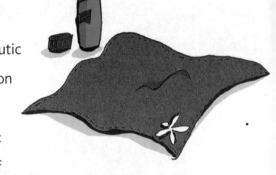

🖐 Carry a handkerchief
moistened with a few drops of lemon or almond essential oil.

🖐 Place a cool lavender-scented compress on your forehead
and a warm compress over your rib cage.

🖐 When you're at home, put three drops of lavender essential
oil and one of peppermint essential oil in a diffuser or humidifier
to scent the air around you.

🖐 Another aromatherapy remedy is to get a massage done
with camomile massage oil.

listen it away

MorningWell (*www.morningwell.com*) is a relatively new audio program created from a unique blend of music, pulses, and specific frequencies to relieve morning sickness, and it has worked for a number of moms. It comes on an audiocassette tape and—when listened to through headphones—is conveyed by the body's vestibular system (a little-known part of our sensory system).

It works by interrupting the passage of signals between the brain and the gut that would normally cause emesis (the urge to vomit).

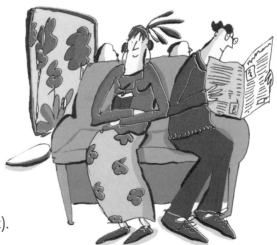

stick out your tongue

This remedy didn't work for me—and I wouldn't recommend it if a gag reflex is your ticket to vomiting—but some mothers swear by it, so here it is. To avoid actually vomiting, try grasping your tongue with a piece of cloth and pulling it gently but firmly.

This is supposed to stop you in an embarrassing moment (rather like catching your nose when you're about to sneeze).

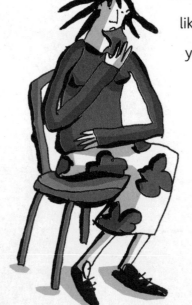

frozen pops

Preggie Pops look pretty good and come in four flavors, depending on what you like during those first few months. Ginger, sour fruits, mint, and lavender flavors (all natural) have been shown to help those who are nauseated. These frozen lollipops give you something to suck on (and, ideally, relieve your nausea), and they can be purchased at *www.morningsicknesshelp.com*.

If you're in the mood, you could make them yourself—a health-food store should have the essential oils required. Frozen treats (*see pages 120–121*) helped me immensely.

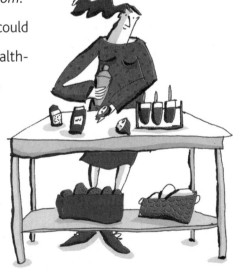

horse pills

During pregnancy, your needs for vitamins B6 and B12, folic acid, zinc, and iron increase. Adequate amounts of these nutrients are probably enough to ward off nausea, but if you are feeling very ill early in your pregnancy, some moms find that extra B6 supplements (around 100 mg daily) are helpful. You may also require B12 (in 50 mcg doses daily) and zinc (aim to have 20 mg daily). Consult your health-care provider to adjust your vitamin dosages in a way that is appropriate for you. On the other hand, some women find that their nausea diminishes if they stop taking their prenatal vitamins or iron supplements temporarily, although you must still take a folic acid supplement to help protect your baby. Iron supplements can be hard for some women to deal with, but if you are reluctant to give them up, try taking them before bed and then, with luck, you will sleep through any nausea.

a few words on meals . . .

To reduce smells when you are cooking, turn on the exhaust fan in your kitchen and/or open a window. I found that taking frequent breaks outside also helped. Using a microwave is a great way to cook without smells (as long as you don't stand in front of it!). Or cook simple foods and let your family know that spices are available and they can flavor their dishes themselves. Avoid spicy and fried food. Cold food (fruit salad, for example) often has fewer nausea-inducing smells associated with it. Don't skip meals if you can help it.

on drinks

If you suffer from heartburn
during pregnancy, avoid having a
lot to drink with meals—you
swallow more air when you
drink while you are eating, and
this can aggravate heartburn

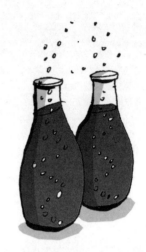

when it subsequently comes up again. Avoid alcohol and drinks
containing caffeine (coffee, tea, cola, *see page 144*) because
these relax the muscle at the top of the stomach holding the
acid in. Instead, try to drink caffeine-free versions of your
favorite drinks or, if you like carbonated drinks, try orange juice
with soda water. You can also add soda water to any other
favorite juice. I started making iced tea out of my favorite
herbal teas, and added lemon and orange juice to it for a little
extra zip (*see page 145*).

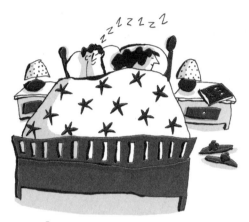

on lying down

When you go to bed, try using a few extra pillows so that you
sleep a bit more upright. Or raise the head of the bed on blocks;
if you and your partner share a heartburn problem, this could be
a great solution for both of you. In bed (or on the couch), lie on
your side as opposed to your back . . . this also helps quell dizzy
spells—for some reason, you seem to get dizzier faster when you
get up from lying on your back. This position also means you can
slide your way to the floor—handy as you get bigger!

antacids

Try taking simple antacid mixtures or tablets. These are available over the counter at the pharmacy and do not contain ingredients that are absorbed, so they cannot harm the baby—they merely neutralize acid in the esophagus and stomach. Avoid indigestion tablets such as cimetidine, ranitidine, and famotidine, which are absorbed into the bloodstream. Eating yogurt or drinking milk can help: their alkaline nature may ease a warring stomach; but cheese can make heartburn worse.

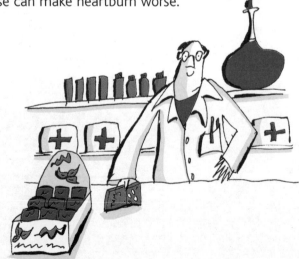

don't slouch

Can you slouch and chew gum at the same time? Sit with good posture when you are eating, for slouching can put extra pressure on your stomach. And to ease heartburn, chew gum or suck on lozenges (not mints) to produce a flow of saliva, which may help control stomach acid. I am the queen of slouchers, so I am not one to talk about good posture. However, when I do manage to sit up straight (like my piano teacher told me), I notice the difference immediately. Good sitting posture also helps ease backache and strengthens those muscles. Avoid lying down or stooping immediately after meals, and if you're having trouble sitting comfortably, place a pillow in the small of your back—this is particularly helpful when you are driving.

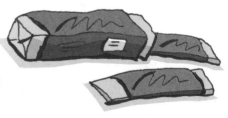

limit your eating before bed

Try not to eat anything in the two or three hours before you go to bed. An empty stomach produces less acid, so you are less likely to have heartburn while you sleep. Of course, this is a beneficial tip only if you aren't suffering from morning sickness and heartburn at the same time! If you want to try a drink, put a tablespoon of honey in a glass of warm milk, for honey is an all-purpose soother. If you don't like the milk idea, place the honey in herbal tea, or even eat it off the spoon.

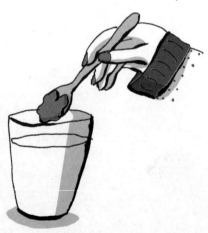

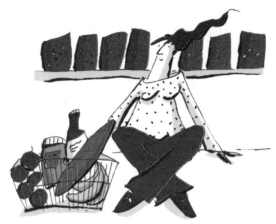

stand out

Avoid standing for long periods of time. This is a good idea for
avoiding leg cramps and varicose veins as well as dizziness.

I found that even if my bout of nausea was over for the day, I
could become light-headed and a bit sweaty while standing in
the checkout line. Always look out for a nearby bench, and don't
be afraid to just sit down in line. One time my dizziness was so
bad that I was afraid I'd black out, so I just plopped down cross-
legged on the floor beside my basket until it passed . . .

take it slowly

When you are sitting, return to a standing position slowly, for getting up too fast can really make you dizzy. While standing, practice contracting and relaxing your leg and buttock muscles to help blood return to your head. I used to rise onto my tiptoes, up and down, to keep the blood moving. And don't get out of a hot bath too quickly. It feels good to lie in the bathtub, but you must take it slowly getting out. If you have trouble as you get bigger, install some temporary handrails on the bathtub to help you keep your balance.

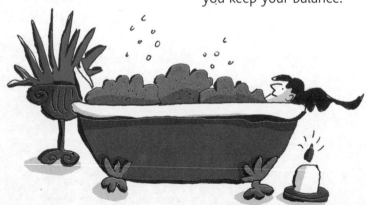

keep cool in hot weather

This is essential to avoid many ailments—swollen feet, heatstroke, and the like. Find a shady place while the kids play in the pool, then drink some cold water and read the day away. Staying still will keep you from getting too hot, even in the sweatiest weather. And make sure that your blood sugar isn't low, by eating small protein-rich snacks throughout the day. Some moms swear that a potassium-rich banana or a milk shake can do wonders.

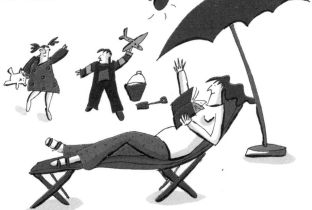

constipation

eat your veggies

Keep plenty of fruit and vegetables in your diet. This goes without saying, but if you are having a problem with constipation, then increasing your intake of a variety of fruit and veggies will help keep things moving. Pick foods you like—don't feel that you have to eat brussels sprouts if you hate them. Buy a box of raisins or a mango instead. And do drink plenty of fluids. Water is your best bet in most situations (*see pages 146–147*), but if you're really having trouble, prune juice is a great solution. Just remember: a little goes a long way.

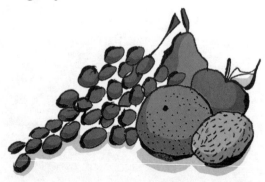

constipation

get moving!

Regular exercise—especially squatting, swimming, and walking—
can relieve constipation. It's more tempting just to sit, but
keeping your body moving (slowly—you don't have to train
for a marathon) will keep your insides moving well. Leg cramps
can also be avoided by taking plenty of exercise.

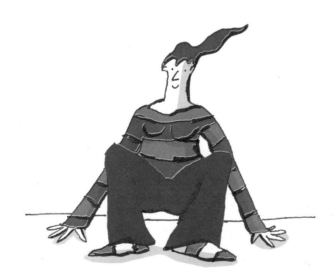

constipation

when you have to go . . . GO

Don't try to hold off for a while (unless of course you're stuck in
a traffic jam, on public transportation, or in a situation where no
bathroom is available)—doing so can cause constipation and,
later on, hemorrhoids (*see pages 54–55*). It is important to
learn to respond to your body, no matter what it is asking of
you. Avoid straining your bowels (another lovely topic, but a
necessary one). Don't sit forever, and don't strain, for this can
only make things worse. If you are having trouble, go for a
little walk and drink some water.

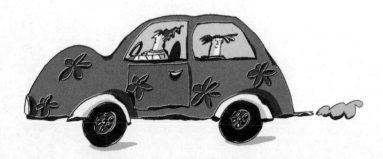

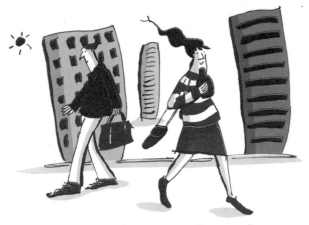

adequate calcium intake

Getting plenty of calcium is important in preventing leg cramps. Three servings every day of yogurt, milk, or cheese can go a long way toward preventing cramps before they start. If you're on the run during the day, several yogurt companies now offer yogurt-on-the-go or yogurt smoothies in plastic bottles for easy drinking. When a cramp begins, flex your toes toward you and massage the muscle slowly. Running your fingers up and down your leg, in a "piano-playing" motion, can also relieve the pain.

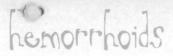

an herbal solution

Comfrey and yellowdock-root ointments are herbal alternatives
to traditional hemorrhoid treatments, which you should be able
to find in cream or ointment form at a health-food store (for
advice on using herbal medicine in pregnancy, *see page 10*). Use
them just as you would Preparation H—they reportedly have a
more soothing effect than commercial ointments. But if you
can't find them, try plain old Preparation H, as it can really help
if you are in a lot of discomfort. Herbal sitz baths are another
great solution if you are particularly tired of ointments and pads,
and just want to relax for a bit. Place herbal tea bags of comfrey
(or primarily comfrey, maybe mixed with camomile) in the bath
with you. A sitz bath should be only two or three inches deep;
if you just want to relax, throw a little baking soda in the bath
with you, and the teabags, and lie back for some soothing relief.

hemorrhoids

a little dab

Apply baking soda wet or dry to take away the itch of
hemorrhoids—you can make up a solution (about two
tablespoons of baking soda to 8 fl oz/225 ml of water) and keep
it in a spray bottle or a cup in the bathroom. Spray or pour a bit
of the solution on some toilet paper, and dab—don't wipe—the
irritated area. Some moms recommend witch hazel or lemon
juice to reduce swelling or bleeding. However, if your
hemorrhoids are bleeding, consult a doctor before
trying home remedies (lemon juice will sting if
they are bleeding, but witch hazel should be fine).
Both can also be dabbed on with toilet paper or
absorbent cotton balls. Tuck's Pads are a
commercially available witch-hazel solution
that come with a pad in the jar.

the funky chicken?

Pelvic rocking is an effective exercise that you'll want to do only when no one else is around! It's the dirty dancing of back-pain relief, but it does help. Stand up straight with your feet shoulder width apart and one leg slightly in front of the other (for balance), then move your pelvic area—keeping your upper body straight—back and forth and around, until your back pain starts to feel better.

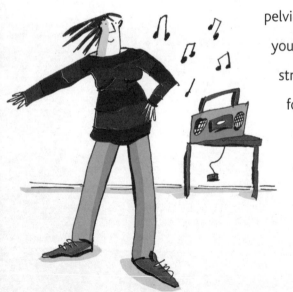

R&R

It's hard to do this yourself, so enlist your partner to massage you; or, if you can afford it, pay someone for 20 minutes of relief. Failing that, roll a tennis ball along your own back or look into purchasing large, flexible exercise balls. They come in different sizes, up to 36 inches (90 cm) in diameter, and you lie with your back on them, pushing yourself back and forth with your feet. Another tip is to sleep on your side, and put a pillow between your knees to reduce the strain. I'm not pregnant anymore and I still do it! Heat also helps, whether it's a bath, a heating pad (on nothing higher than medium, and only on your back), or a hot water bottle. And I found that heat inserts, sold by stores for hunters to put in their boots or gloves, were good for long car rides.

those flat-heeled shoes

Wear flat-heeled shoes that offer good support. It's tough to be fashionable and pregnant, and shoes are one area where comfort must come first during your pregnant months. Try to get away with sneakers as much as possible, but if you are working and need to look professional, buy flats. If they don't have good support, buy some gel inserts to help you out.

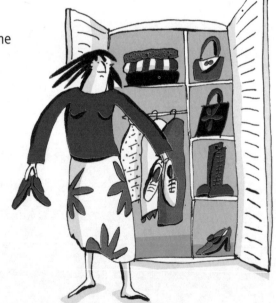

the everlasting cold

Ah, the ever-present pregnancy cold. Here are some ways other moms have suggested to get through the coughing, sneezing, aching days. Increase your intake of vitamin C foods: an orange before bedtime, some rosehip tea at lunch . . . any food rich in vitamin C may help prevent colds—and ease them once you've 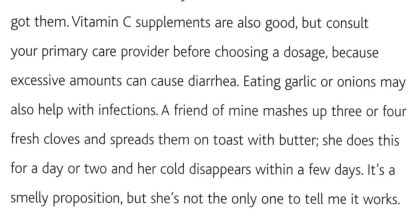 got them. Vitamin C supplements are also good, but consult your primary care provider before choosing a dosage, because excessive amounts can cause diarrhea. Eating garlic or onions may also help with infections. A friend of mine mashes up three or four fresh cloves and spreads them on toast with butter; she does this for a day or two and her cold disappears within a few days. It's a smelly proposition, but she's not the only one to tell me it works.

clear the air

Keeping the air moist can help to relieve cold symptoms and keep you breathing freely. Eucalyptus, lavender, lemon, and tea tree make a good combination for congestion: put two drops of each essential oil into a bowl of hot water, then place a towel over your head and inhale the steam for 10 minutes. However, do not use this remedy in conjunction with homeopathic remedies.

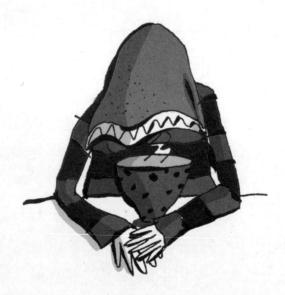

an herbal decoction

One mom suggested this hot decoction as a useful cold remedy:
cloves have antiseptic and stimulant qualities, coriander seeds
aid digestion, honey is soothing to the throat, and ginger is
soothing to the stomach.

ingredients

For a pitcher of herbal tea, you need: 4 cloves; 1 tsp coriander seeds;
a few slices of fresh ginger; 1 pt (600 ml) water; slice of lemon; honey

Put the cloves, coriander seeds, and fresh ginger in the water, then
bring to a boil and simmer for 20 minutes. Add a slice of lemon and
simmer for an additional 5 minutes. Strain and sweeten with honey
to taste. Drink a hot cup of this decoction every two hours.

cold tea

You can drink this cold tea as often as necessary to relieve cold symptoms. Fresh leaves are best, although dried ones are easiest to use with a strainer.

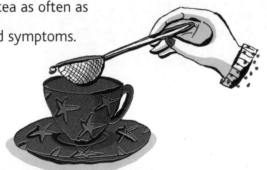

ingredients

You need: equal parts of peppermint, chickweed, echinacea, and blackberry leaves; empty tea bags (from any health-food store, or use a piece of fine cheesecloth); boiling water; honey to taste

Mix the leaves in a container, then put a heaping teaspoon into a tea bag. Steep in boiling water for 10 minutes; sweeten as desired.

insomnia

Sure, you can't sleep now, but wait until the baby is born ... Here are some tips to help you get the rest you need now. Avoid stimulants and eat a few hours before bedtime, making sure that your meal is easily digestible. Also ensure that your room is well ventilated and that your bed is comfortable; massage of the head and neck before bed may relieve tension. But don't assume that all sleep must be gotten at night. A good nap of 20–90 minutes (no more) can do wonders, especially between 1 p.m. and 3 p.m. Studies have shown that those who take naps often sleep longer and harder at night.

exercise

Exercise? You mean I have to carry this baby around
all the time and exercise, too? Isn't doing the laundry
and the dishes, and going to work every day enough?
Well, yes and no. Doing chores is a great way to keep in
shape—and if you're like me and get bored easily with
walking on the treadmill, then doing the housework with
some extra "oomph" might be all you need. But there are
many exercises that can help you to relax and that can
soothe any worries you may be facing in pregnancy.

Moderate exercise keeps your muscles strong and
flexible, which will be useful during labor. It also reduces
the physical discomforts of pregnancy, such as backache

exercise

and constipation, and makes getting your body back into shape after childbirth that much easier. But don't forget: there are limits on what exercise you can do, now that you're pregnant —your center of gravity has shifted, you're carrying more weight, and you tire more quickly. That's why you must follow expert advice, exercise with care, and listen closely to what your body is telling you. It will often warn you when you're pushing it too hard.

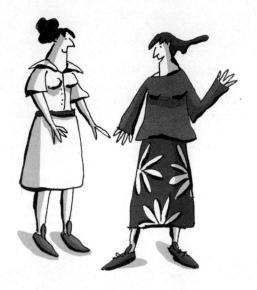

listen to the professionals

Check with your doctor or midwife before starting an exercise program. If you have always been active, you can probably continue your existing exercise regime provided your pregnancy isn't considered high risk, but check that the activities you participate in are right for you. If you've never been the athletic type, he or she can give you some helpful tips on getting started.

what to wear

Wear loose-fitting, breathable clothing and supportive shoes. To avoid overheating while you exercise, layer clothes so that they're easy to remove, or wear outfits specially designed for exercise. And make sure your maternity bra offers enough support. You'll also need athletic shoes that fit your feet properly, to help support the ligaments and tendons. If your shoe size has changed because of mild swelling, buy a new, comfortable pair.

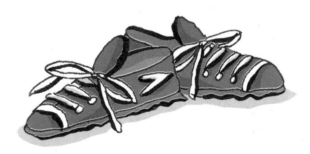

warm up before exercising

Warm-ups do just that—they warm up your muscles and joints to prepare your body for exercise, and help build your heart rate up slowly. If you skip the warm-up and jump into strenuous activity before your body is ready, you could strain your ligaments and hurt yourself. And keep moving while you exercise: change positions frequently or walk on the spot. Standing motionless for prolonged stretches, which certain yoga and dance positions call for, can decrease the blood flow to your uterus and cause blood to pool in your legs, making you feel dizzy.

some dos

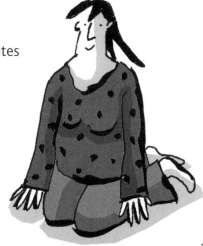 Do stop exercising immediately if you feel uncomfortable or are in pain.

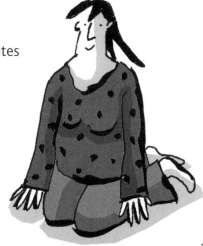 Do listen to your body: when something hurts, something's wrong. You should feel as if you're working your body, not punishing it.

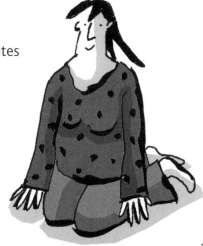 Do get up from the floor slowly and carefully, since getting up quickly can make you dizzy, or might cause you to lose your footing and fall.

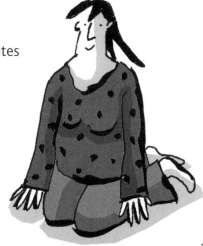 Do cool down afterward by walking in place for a few minutes or stretching. This gives your heart a chance to return gradually to its normal rate.

exercise

some don'ts

🖐 Don't exercise while flat on your back after the first trimester. Besides being uncomfortable, this position can cause dizziness, so rest on your elbows instead, or lie on your side.

🖐 Don't do deep knee bends, lunges, or full sit-ups, because these positions can cause ligament strain and increase the chance of tearing in the pelvic area. Instead, switch to other activities that tone the same muscles: swimming and walking will work the quadriceps and buttock areas just as well as lunges and knee bends.

🖐 Don't overdo it by going for the "burn," and don't exercise to the point of exhaustion: your heart rate shouldn't exceed 140 beats per minute. A good rule of thumb is to slow down if you can't comfortably carry on a conversation.

too hot?

Try to avoid outdoor activities when it's hot and humid.
Pregnant or not, you must take it easy when the sun is blazing
down and the air is as humid as a thick, wet blanket—weather
like this makes you prone to overheating. On particularly hot
or humid days, skip your workout and take it easy, or exercise
indoors in a well-ventilated room.

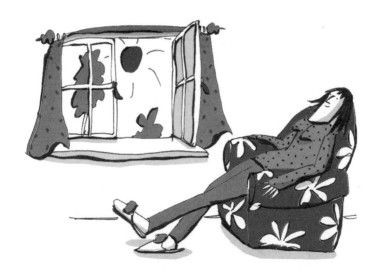

cut out high-risk sports

It might sound obvious, but you'd be surprised . . . Steer clear of dangerous sports. Because your joints are looser than normal, it's best to avoid any activity that could make you slip or fall. Horseback riding, downhill skiing, mountain climbing, and most contact sports (football, basketball, and soccer) are not recommended for you now. Racket sports such as tennis and squash are best avoided, too, because the side-to-side movements can be hard on the knees, and the ball could hit your abdomen at whiplash speed.

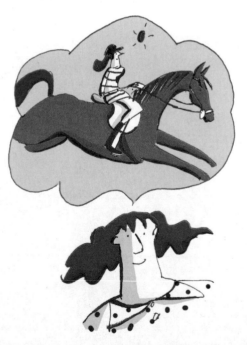

watch for unusual symptoms

If you have any unusual symptoms while exercising, call your midwife or doctor immediately. Although some women experience light spotting throughout their pregnancy, vaginal bleeding is a cause for concern and should be checked out by a professional.

A sharp pain in the abdomen and chest may simply mean that your ligaments are stretching, but you could also be having contractions. If your eyesight gets blurred in the middle of exercising, you may be dehydrated, or you might have pre-eclampsia (*see pages 244–245*), a condition that can be risky for a developing baby. If you have any doubts, do get your symptoms checked out.

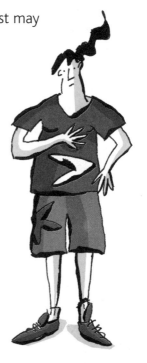

other points to look for

🖐 Whether you're in the middle of pregnancy exercise class or not, fainting may mean that you have a medical problem, and it needs to be checked out.

🖐 Feeling sick means that you may have built up too much lactic acid in your stomach.

🖐 Persistent dizziness, or dizziness that is accompanied by blurred vision and headaches or palpitations, may be a symptom of severe anemia or some other illness that could affect your pregnancy.

🖐 If, while you exercise, you're so breathless that you can't keep up a conversation, you experience any strange, fluttery sensations in your chest, or you sweat buckets, you're probably working too hard, so make sure you are exercising within your safe heart rate range. Slow down gradually and stop; get checked over by your midwife or doctor.

going up?

Have you been horrified to notice increased swelling in your hands, feet, and ankles? Do you feel like an overblown balloon at these points? Your feet and hands may puff up a little after exercise, but if you notice more swelling than usual, it may be an indication of the condition known as pre-eclampsia (*see pages 244–245*), so visit your midwife or doctor as soon as possible for reassurance or for treatment.

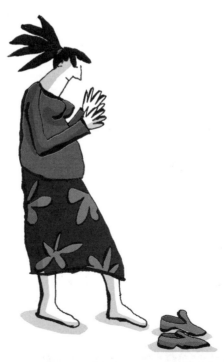

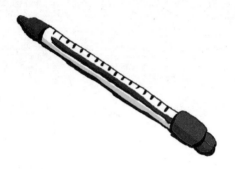

changes in body temperature

If your hands turn clammy, or you get hot or cold flashes, your body is telling you that it's having a hard time regulating its internal thermometer. Your baby can get overheated, just as you do, and blood flowing to the uterus will be diverted to the skin as the body tries to cool itself off, possibly putting the baby in jeopardy. According to the experts, your temperature (when taken under the arm) should be less than 101°F (38.3°C) after exercising, so keep a close eye on this.

watch the clock

It's a tough call: exercise too little and you won't make any progress; exercise too much and you can really harm yourself. So a full workout for a pregnant mom who does light to moderate exercise on a regular basis (and has been approved for working out by her health-care provider) should last about 30–60 minutes, from warm-up to cooldown, in one day. The American

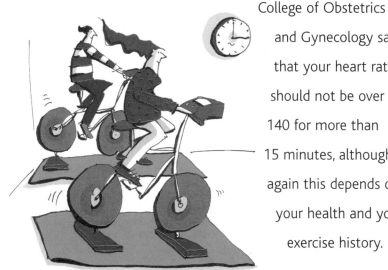

College of Obstetrics and Gynecology says that your heart rate should not be over 140 for more than 15 minutes, although again this depends on your health and your exercise history.

exercise

it's not for everyone

Keep in mind that exercise isn't safe for all pregnant women.
Those who have experienced preterm labor; who have obstetrical
complications (including persistent vaginal bleeding,
incompetent cervix, ruptured membranes, or an indication
that the fetus is not growing as quickly as he or she should);
who have been put on bed rest throughout the term of their
pregnancy; or who have a history of
medical problems (such as high
blood pressure, diabetes, heart
disease, and thyroid disease)—
should exercise *only* with
their doctor's approval.

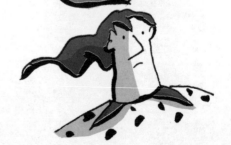

don't exercise to lose weight

You'll certainly gain less fat weight during your pregnancy if you continue to exercise (assuming you exercised before becoming pregnant), but don't expect or try to lose weight by doing so. For most women, the goal is to maintain their fitness level throughout pregnancy. If you are obsessed with your weight and get depressed after every monthly weigh-in, stop looking at the scale. Ask the nurses not to tell you how much you weigh, unless there is a medical reason to do so. And don't even think about going on a diet now. Focus on nutritious eating habits, rather than on the scale: what it says you weigh is not an absolute anyway, since your body undergoes rapid fluid shifts during the day.

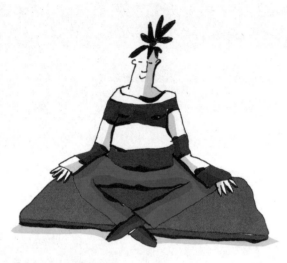

yoga benefits

I am not an expert (or even an amateur) in yoga, but enough
moms told me about the benefits of yoga to a pregnant mother
and her child that I thought I should include it here. Yoga stretches
(a few of which are given on the following pages) help to keep
the body supple and enhance good posture; for moms-to-be,
they can help to promote a relatively trouble-free pregnancy
and childbirth by working gently on the reproductive organs and

pelvis and helping to ensure that the growing fetus receives a good supply of blood and nutrients. Those who haven't previously done yoga poses (*asanas*) should be particularly careful during the first three months of pregnancy, although breathing and relaxation exercises will generally be beneficial; after the third month, it should be safe to start practicing gentle yoga poses. As always, listen to your body and stop if it tells you to do so.

Yoga breathing exercises (*pranayama*) increase the lungs' capacity, encouraging an abundant supply of oxygen to your child, and help prepare you for labor. Meditation can alleviate many of the aches and worries that are common in pregnancy, and enable you to connect with your developing child. Hand gestures (*mudras*) and locks (*bandhas*) can have powerful effects on a woman's reproductive organs. And deep relaxation (*yoga nidra*) is soothing—both physically and mentally—during pregnancy.

churning-the-mill pose

This pose is useful for preparing your abdomen for pregnancy, and also makes a great postnatal exercise.

Sit on the floor with your legs straight out in front of you and 12 inches (30 cm) or so apart. Lock the fingers of both hands together and hold them straight out in front of you. Now make sweeping circles with your hands over your feet, learning as far forward as possible and then as far back as possible. Repeat the exercise 10 times in each direction.

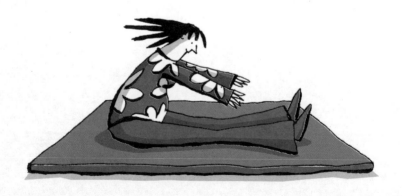

palm tree pose

A backache is a never-ending issue in pregnancy and, even though I didn't know it was yoga, I've done this exercise many times. It relieves back pain and helps with posture.

Stand upright with your feet together and your arms resting loosely by your sides. Lift your arms over your head, place the palms of your hands together, entwine your fingers, then turn your palms so that they face upward. Straighten your elbows, then stretch your whole body upward as you stand on tiptoe and breathe in. Lower your heels to the floor and breathe out, placing your hands on your head. Relax for a while, then repeat the sequence up to 10 times.

flapping fish pose

The flapping fish pose is excellent for relieving constipation and relaxing the nerves in the legs and back. Once again, this was an exercise that I did without knowing it was a yoga move, and it relieved my sciatica immensely. You can support your knee and head on pillows, if you wish.

Lie on your front, then turn slightly to bend your right knee up toward your chest, keeping the other leg straight on the floor. Place your right elbow either on your right knee or on the floor (whichever is more comfortable), and the left side of your head on your left arm. Relax for a while, then repeat on the other side.

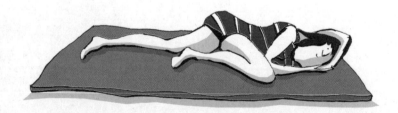

(gentle) ankle crank

This is another great exercise that's just as much common sense as it is yoga. It helps the circulation in your legs and feet.

While sitting down, bend your left knee and bring your left foot up to rest on your right knee. Holding your left toes in your right hand, and your left ankle with your left hand, gently rotate the ankle in as wide a circle as possible. Perform 10 rotations clockwise and 10 rotations counterclockwise, then repeat the exercise with the other ankle.

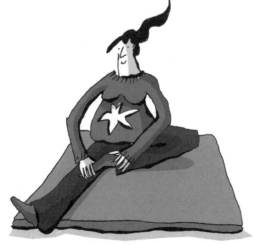

half butterfly pose

A great exercise for loosening up the hip joints and the legs is the half butterfly, although it's important that you not strain yourself to achieve this pose.

Sit on the floor with your legs straight out in front of you. Bending your left leg, position your left foot on your right thigh, as high up as you can. Then put your left hand on your left knee and grasp the toes of your left foot in your right hand. Inhale as you pull your left knee up toward your chest; exhale as you push your knee down toward the floor, ensuring that any movement is created by pressure of your left arm, rather than by moving your body. Repeat the process 10 times with each leg.

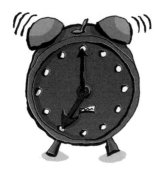

a little means a lot

If you've been relatively inactive before your pregnancy, then now is not the time to start a major workout plan. Start slowly and build up gradually. Find some form of exercise that you like (or a couple of different activities), and do them at your own pace. If your body begins to scream "Stop!"—then do so. Five minutes of exercise is better than none at all, and if you are consistent, you'll find that you are better able to exercise for longer periods of time.

exercise with a friend

Exercising with a friend—even if it's only going on a walk together—is a great way to catch up on news and exercise at the same time. One woman, who hadn't exercised pre-pregnancy, said that she lived down the road from a senior center and started walking with an older woman every day. She made an instant friend and found that they both walked at the same pace!

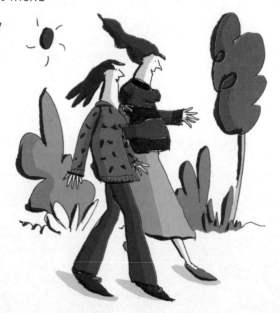

check out the mall

I was between eight and nine months pregnant with my second child during the hottest time of the year. I was miserable: my feet and ankles swelled—sometimes so much that I couldn't get my feet into my slip-on shoes—and I felt big and sweaty all the time. I found that one of the best places for me to retreat to was the local, air-conditioned mall. Not only could I cool off there, but I actually felt like walking around and getting a bit of exercise—provided of course that I could actually get my feet into my shoes before I left!

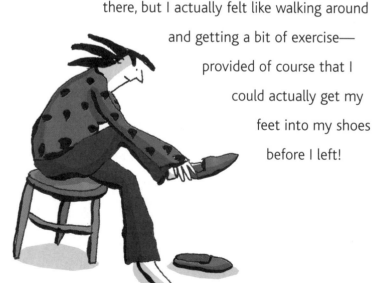

drink lots of water

It is extremely important to stay well hydrated before,
during, and after exercise—at all times, but particularly
throughout your pregnancy. If you don't drink plenty of fluids,
you can become dehydrated, which may cause contractions
and raise your body temperature. Many people swear by sports
drinks, like Gatorade, but plain old water is just fine. Get into the
habit of keeping a bottle of water with you at all times (just in
case you get the urge to walk around!) and fill it up before you
leave the house. You need to drink about two glasses of water
two hours before you begin exercising, then another glass or
two every 15–20 minutes during your workout.

If you are going to be gone from the house for the day,
one mom recommends putting a bottle of water in the freezer
overnight, then taking it with you the next day: by midday, it
will have thawed sufficiently for you to drink it. Getting into

exercise

the habit of having water with you all the time will also serve you well once your baby arrives, because a hungry, always-nursing baby tends to make mama very thirsty!

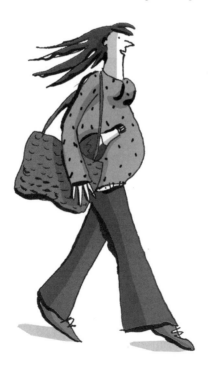

kegels

This exercise (named after the doctor who supposedly invented it) involves alternately contracting and releasing the muscles of the pelvic floor and birth canal. Contracting the muscles supports the abdomen and internal organs (especially necessary after you have had children), and relaxing them teaches you how to let go so that the baby can pass through the birth canal.

Sit upright on a firm chair, making sure that your weight is resting on the two rocker-like bones (the "sits bones") on either side of your vagina and that you're not slumped on your tailbone; try to squeeze the muscles between your sits bones and lift them up inside. Hold for 10 seconds (but keep breathing!), then slowly relax the muscles, noticing how they fall toward the surface of the chair. Start with five repetitions, then work up to 10, two or three times a day.

c curves

To relieve low backache in pregnancy and labor, and to help ease the baby's passage through the birth canal, try the following exercise, which works on the deep abdominal muscles and curves the lumbar spine (at the back of the waist) into a C shape.

Sit upright on a firm chair, relax your abdomen, and breathe in; then breathe out, tightening your deep abdominal muscles and rolling back slightly onto your tailbone, so that your lumbar spine makes the desired C shape. Now relax your chest and shoulders; breathe in and return to an upright position. Do 10 repetitions, two or three times a day.

get help

If you have previously been very active and there are no medical complications, you can continue to be so, although you need to modify your activities; this is where a good pre/post-natal fitness specialist can be a great help. If you have not been active and are less than 26 weeks along, find a specialist who is certified to teach group classes; you will gain from the activity and from the group support. If you are more than 26 weeks, get qualified advice: there are still many health benefits to be had for mom and baby, and endurance training is a big help in labor. Dos: aerobic dancing, walking, swimming, stationary cycling, low-impact aerobics. Don'ts: high-step aerobics, scuba diving, and competitive team sports.

exercise

relax

Relaxation provides important benefits for body and mind, and can renew your energy and enhance your experience of the life growing within you. Relaxing on your side maximizes blood flow to the uterus, which is beneficial for your baby. So find a quiet place and lie down on your side, with your knees, hips, shoulders, and elbows slightly bent; make yourself comfortable with pillows. Breathe slowly and deeply. Focus on an image of your baby growing healthy and strong. Listening to peaceful music can be very helpful. Do this for 10–20 minutes each day.

squatting

Squatting strengthens the upper thighs and opens the birth
outlet, but if you have knee or other joint problems, don't do it.

From a seated position, place one foot flat on the floor with the
knee of that leg deeply bent; lean your weight onto both hands,
which should be placed forward and slightly to the other side.
Now put your other foot flat onto the floor. Keep your weight
comfortably distributed among the four supports, and relax your
bottom. To get out of the squat, reverse the process.

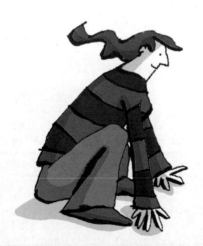

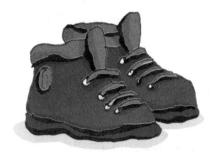

walking

🖐 In the first trimester, you won't need to stray too far from your normal walking habits, but do make sure you have proper walking shoes so that your feet get the support they need. If it's hot and humid outside, skip the walk entirely.

🖐 Second trimester: you may now feel more ungainly, so pay attention to your posture when you walk, to avoid straining your back. Keep your head straight, chin level, hips tucked under your shoulders (to avoid arching your back), and eyes on whatever lies ahead. Swing your arms for balance and to intensify your workout.

🖐 Third trimester: keep doing what you have been for as long as you can, but avoid uneven terrain that could put you off-balance.

jogging

✋ Follow the usual precautions in the first trimester, such as monitoring your heart rate and drinking lots of water before, during, and after a jog. Avoid running in hot and humid weather, and wear proper shoes that offer plenty of support for your feet.

✋ Second trimester: your center of gravity is shifting now, leaving you vulnerable to slips and falls. For safety, stick to flat pavements. If you do lose your balance, try to fall correctly—sideways or onto your hands and knees, rather than directly onto your abdomen.

✋ Third trimester: be just as careful as you've been in the first two trimesters. And remember: if you feel too fatigued to go for a run, listen to your body and take a break. Pushing yourself too hard may be harmful.

exercise

swimming

🖐 If energy levels permit, swim for at least 20 minutes every other day in the first trimester, for maximum benefit. Swimming first thing in the morning may counteract morning sickness.

🖐 Second trimester: your pregnancy won't require you to cut down on swimming as you grow, since it's easy on expectant mothers—the water supports your joints and ligaments as you exercise, preventing injury, and protects you from overheating.

🖐 Third trimester: a maternity swimsuit may be necessary now. Look out for local antenatal/aquanatal exercise classes.

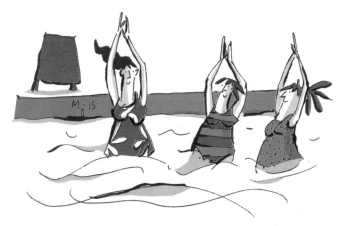

get pumped

Weight training will help prepare you for lifting an increasingly heavy infant. If you haven't previously done any strength work, get assistance from someone who is qualified to teach a pregnant woman. You should be aiming to move a weight or resistance until your muscle begins to fatigue. One mom says that a simple way to start at home is to carry 1-lb (450-g) or 2-lb (900-g) food cans while you take a 10-minute walk at a brisk pace.

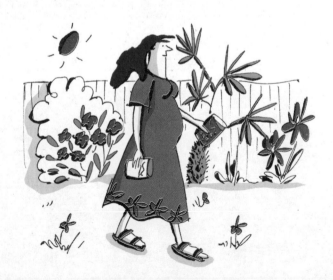

if you weight-train already . . .

🖐 During the first trimester, you can probably continue your regular routine, but pay attention to your technique. Use slow, controlled movements to lift weights, rather than relying on momentum to hoist them up. This will avoid injury to your joints, which are loosened by the pregnancy hormone relaxin.

🖐 Second trimester: you should now avoid lifting weights while standing up. The blood-vessel walls are affected by the hormones produced in pregnancy, so you are more prone to varicose veins and pooling of blood in the lower limbs. This could leave you feeling light-headed and dizzy, so sit down to weight-train.

🖐 Third trimester: you don't need to take any additional precautions during the third trimester, but do make sure you inform your health-care practitioner that you are weight training.

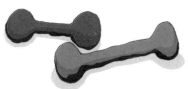

military press

Sit up straight on the edge of a sturdy chair, with your knees
bent and your feet flat on the floor and about hip width apart.
Hold a dumbbell (weighing 1–5 lb/0.5–2.25 kg) in each hand.
With your palms facing inward, lift the weights
above shoulder level (either one at a time
or both together) and then back down
to shoulder height. Keep the number
of reps low, take a rest, then do
another set. This exercise works
your triceps but remember to
contract your abdominal muscles
and squeeze your shoulder blades
together, and breathe rhythmically.
Tip: if you need more support, sit
back on your chair seat.

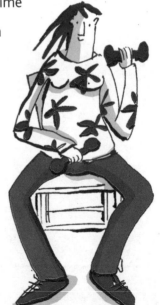

seated row

Sit erect on the floor, with your legs straight out in front of you and knees slightly bent. Wrap a resistance band around both of your feet and hold one end in each hand. Keep your elbows bent close to your sides, with your palms facing each other. Pull the band toward your waist, using your middle back muscles, until your elbows are just behind you. Remember to contract your abdominal muscles and squeeze your shoulder blades together, and breathe rhythmically. Tip: don't lean forward. If you need to increase the resistance, do so by "choking up" on the band—that is, reaching up higher on it and closer to your feet. Sit in front of a chair or sofa for extra support.

dancing

You can get your heart pumping by dancing to your favorite tunes in the comfort of your living room, but steer clear of movements that call for you to leap, jump, or twirl. Remember: technique is important, and there are a number of tips that should help you avoid stressing your joints. Avoid sudden directional changes at speed. Keep your pelvis stable and centered when doing scoops

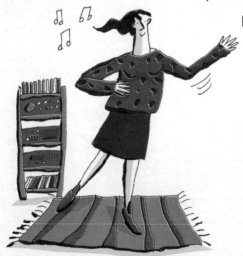

(no funky moves!). Keep your hips level and your abdomen pulled in when doing knee lifts. Avoid knee lifts with high arms (parachute pulls), especially when moving around the room, as they strain your lower back.

taking classes

If you sign up for a class, you can lose yourself in music, stay fit, and meet others. In theory, you can also stay fit at home with the help of an exercise video, but it's best if you choose a class designed for expectant mothers: you'll enjoy the company of other women in the same boat as you, and can rest assured that the instructor is qualified to adapt the exercises to the needs of moms-to-be. If you already attend a regular aerobics class, let the instructor know you're pregnant; he or she can then suggest ways to modify movements.

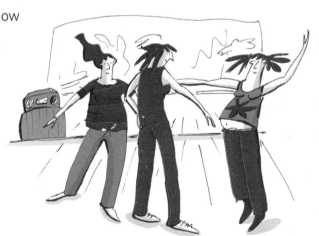

exercise

flying arm exercise

This exercise helps to increase the
flow of blood, stretching the
back (thus reducing back
strain for pregnant
moms) and aiding
relaxation and stress relief.

Raise your arms over your
head, keeping your elbows straight
and the palms of your hands
facing each other. Hold
this position for at least
20 seconds, then lower your
arms out to the sides, keeping your upper back straight. Now
bring the backs of your hands together, as far as possible behind
your back, and stretch. Repeat the whole process five times.

abdominal muscles

During pregnancy, your abdominal muscles will soften, but it is important to check for separation of the abdominal muscles, which can increase your back pain significantly, as these muscles are required to control pelvis tilt and posture. To check for separation: lie on your back and bend your knees, with your feet flat on the floor. Slowly lift your chin toward your chest, raising your head and shoulders until your neck is 6–8 inches (15–20 cm) from the floor. Hold one arm out in front of you; with the other hand, check for a gap (usually present in the first few months of pregnancy or postpartum) or a bulge (in the last three months of pregnancy) in the middle of your abdomen. If any separation is found, cross your hands over your abdominal area to support and "knit" the muscles together. Exhale as you lift your head; this decreases pressure in your abdomen. Avoid abdominal bulging by contracting your abdominal muscle when lifting, and avoid straining of any kind.

pelvic tilt

This exercise is important—it is the building block of good posture, and it strengthens your abdominal and back muscles, thereby decreasing back strain and fatigue. Practice it often.

Lie on your back with your knees bent. Breathe in through your nose, and tighten your stomach and buttock muscles. Flatten the small of your back against the floor and let your pelvis (your hip bones and sacrum) tilt upward. Hold for a count of five as you exhale slowly. Relax, then repeat. You can also perform the pelvic tilt while on your hands and knees or while standing upright. *Caution*: do not arch your back, bulge your abdomen, or push with your feet to achieve the tilt.

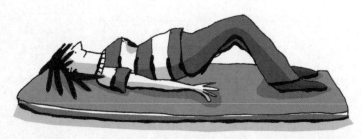

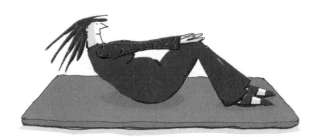

sit-ups

Gentle sit-ups can prevent a lot of back pain later on—a lesson
I learned the hard way by not doing them! There are two variations.

🖐 For the forward sit-up, lie on your back with your knees bent
and breathe in slowly through your nose. Breathe out through
partially pursed lips as you raise your head, with hands pointing to
your knees or behind your head. Lift your chin toward your chest
and lift your shoulders off the floor (but not more than 45°).

🖐 For the diagonal sit-up, lie down as before. Point your right
hand toward your left knee while raising your head and right
shoulder. Breathe out slowly through your mouth. Keep your
left knee slightly bent and your left heel on the floor.

calf stretch

This is a good exercise for moms-to-be to do before going to bed if you are bothered by leg cramps at night, which can be quite painful and make you feel as though you have been kicked by a mule!

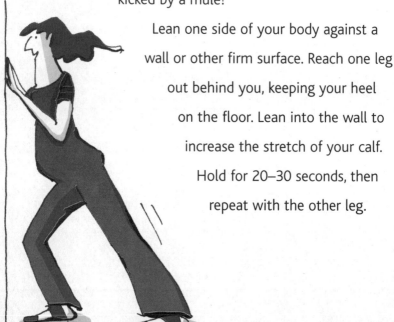

Lean one side of your body against a wall or other firm surface. Reach one leg out behind you, keeping your heel on the floor. Lean into the wall to increase the stretch of your calf. Hold for 20–30 seconds, then repeat with the other leg.

don't "work out"

Working out is hard. I, for one, am not the
kind of person who is going to wake up
at 5 a.m. and go to the gym.
I might fantasize that I am, but
I'm not. However, I am the kind
of person who will take a walk
after dinner, or sprint up the hill in
my backyard a few times after getting the mail (I have a long
driveway). Figure out what it is that will get you going: you don't
have to pump iron. I have hardwood floors on every level of my
house, and if I take one hour to sweep and mop all the floors,
I feel like I've just spent 30 minutes on the treadmill. Mowing
the lawn (with a push mower!), vacuuming for 15–20 minutes,
riding your bike to the local store for the paper every day—these
are all great ways to exercise and yet not have to "work out."

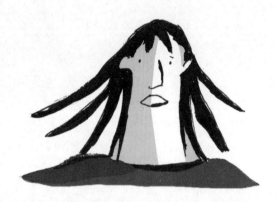

prepare for the birth

Gaining control over your breathing can help you manage pain, and in the event of a lengthy labor, increased endurance may be of real assistance. By practicing breathing in through your nose and out through your mouth in various forms of exercise, from walking to stretching, you are learning how to breathe through the strain of labor.

breech exercises

Do breech exercises (to turn the baby for a normal headfirst delivery) really work? Well, certified nurse-midwife Peg Plumbo says they may. "There is some evidence that breech exercises do work, but because most babies turn spontaneously before 34 weeks, it is hard to substantiate this . . . Breech exercises generally involve positioning yourself so that your buttocks are elevated above your head. Some women lie on an ironing board, which is gently inclined with one end on a couch and the other end on the floor. Lying in this position for 20 minutes, three times a day, might give the baby the message that it should turn around, but if you become nauseated or light-headed do not continue this exercise. I hope this works for you, but in most cases the baby will reposition itself without any special regime."

what to eat

Although it's true that in those first few months you

should eat what you feel like eating, particularly if you're

suffering from extreme nausea, you do need to bear good

nutritional rules in mind all through your pregnancy. You

do not always need to eat enough for two people, but

remember that everything you put in your mouth goes to

your baby and helps form his brain cells, spinal cord, and

those 10 fingers and toes you want to see when he's born.

There are a lot of food choices out there, and you

want to maximize yours by getting what's best for you and

your baby. Don't worry—this isn't a lecture on why you

should never touch another chocolate bar. Look at this

what to eat

chapter as a way to have your chocolate bar and still eat correctly. These tips are not aimed at making eating in pregnancy a miserable, restrictive experience, but rather at helping you find the most beneficial food—and enjoying it.

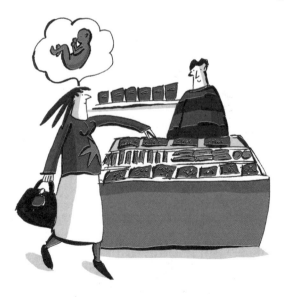

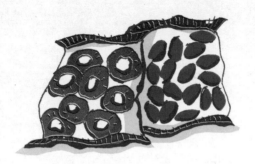

change your habits

You might think it will be difficult to change your eating habits, but I found that, because things were already altering so much in my body, changing my eating habits was just another item on the list. You can let go of a sweet tooth by simply quitting "cold turkey"—it's actually easiest to stop eating sugar altogether, because having a little bit always leads to wanting some more. And look at what you're about to put inside you: will it be beneficial to your baby? If you're pressed for time, keep some dry fruit or a granola bar in a bag to grab on the way to work.

time and money

Time and money are two of the most common reasons for not eating—or not eating well—and they are cop-outs! Fruits and vegetables are far less expensive than prepackaged meals and convenience foods. One apple or one orange at the market costs less than a quarter, whereas a bag of chips is 99 cents! Grab the fruit instead. As for time? You can eat that apple in the car on the way to a meeting, or even as you're walking down the street; you can also eat granola bars, trail mix, yogurt, and a wide variety of other healthful foods on the run.

coping with cravings

Give in to your urge for pickles. One of the causes of morning sickness is low sodium in the blood, which pickles help to replace; and the dill in pickles may be soothing to the intestinal tract. Many pregnant women crave ginger products, which can help nausea; but avoid concentrated ginger supplements, because high doses may be harmful to the fetus—discuss your dosage with your health-care provider if you have any concerns. Instead, drink ginger tea (*see page 35*) and eat gingery Asian food. Cravings for

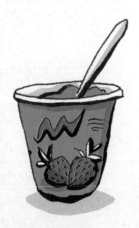

sweets often occur because of a drop in blood sugar levels. To prevent this, eat regular meals and snacks, including plenty of whole grains. Eat sweets that have some nutritional content, such as frozen fruit pops, low-fat vanilla or fruit-flavored yogurts, and chocolate milk.

prenatal supplements

Take a prenatal supplement every day. It provides the vitamins and minerals you need, such as folic acid, iron, zinc, iodine, vitamin D, calcium, and vitamin A. However, unless advised otherwise, you should avoid taking straight vitamin A supplements, or more than the recommended daily amount— 5,000 international units—of vitamin A (which is found in liver and liver products, including liver pâté), because large amounts of this vitamin may be harmful to pregnant women and can cause birth defects.

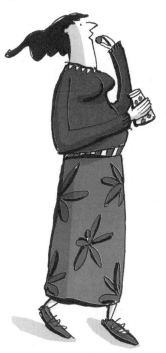

banana smoothies

"I don't know about anyone else," one mom says, "but I find myself craving frozen foods. Here are two recipes I've made up that turned out really well—and they're pretty good for you, too." This recipe for banana smoothies offers lots of protein, calcium, and B vitamins—and it's easy on the tummy.

ingredients

For two banana smoothies, you need: 1 banana; 2 cups milk or soy milk; handful of almonds; 4 ice cubes

Cut up the banana and freeze it. Place in a container, then cover with the milk or soy milk, the almonds, and ice cubes. Blend till smooth.

sweet pumpkin pops

And here's the other frozen recipe: pumpkin contains lots of vitamin A and is a great food for vegetarians; the spice peps it up and brings out its flavor.

ingredients

For 4–6 pops, you need: 2 packages vanilla instant-pudding mix; $2/3$ cup low-fat or skim milk; 1 can solid-pack pumpkin; 1 tub fat-free Cool Whip (or whipping cream); pumpkin-pie spice to taste

Mix the instant pudding with the milk, then stir in the other ingredients and pour into paper or plastic cups. Freeze for $1/2$–1 hour, then insert Popsicle sticks in the middle and freeze for another 3 hours or so. To release the pops from the cups, run hot tap water over the outside for a few seconds, then ease them out.

weight watching

First of all, don't stress out about it! If you eat normally, you shouldn't gain too much weight. To get some idea: moms-to-be need to consume just 300 extra calories a day to support their baby's development (the equivalent of a cup of yogurt and a piece of fruit). Women of normal weight should gain 25–35 lb (11–15 kg); overweight women just 15–25 lb (7–11 kg). Water is responsible for nearly 62 percent of the weight gained by pregnant mothers; 30 percent is from fat and 8 percent from protein. It is important, then, to be careful when choosing your foods. Select lean meats such as fish and chicken (without the skin). Eat eggs, yogurt, or cottage cheese instead of peanut butter, and put skim milk in your coffee or tea.

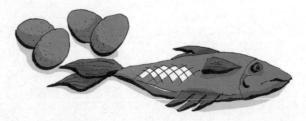

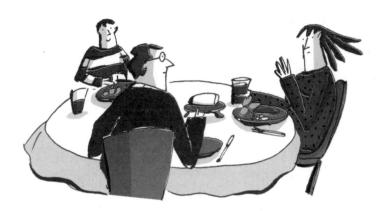

going up?

If you're gaining weight too fast and you'd like to slow your rate of increase (don't try to stop it altogether!), or if your health-care provider suggests that you cut back, first stop looking at your weight. Then cut down on your fat intake—this is the only nutritional requirement that it is safe to restrict. So, no butter on your bread, no oil on your salad, and try to eliminate fried foods altogether.

twins: extra milk

Compared with a woman carrying only one baby, pregnant moms who are having twins need to eat an additional 500–1,000 calories per day, and get an additional ¾ oz (20 g) of protein, beginning at about 20 weeks gestation. In all, you need about 3–4 oz (85–115 g) of protein daily. You will also need more vitamins and minerals, particularly iron, so you should ensure you are taking a daily prenatal vitamin.

One of the best ways for you to get your additional protein is by drinking more milk. This is not only a good source of high-quality protein, but also contains the calcium your babies will need. One cup of milk will give you about 8 g of protein. According to *Nutrition for a Healthy Pregnancy* by leading nutritionist Elizabeth Somers, a woman who is carrying twins should get the equivalent of six glasses of milk per day. But although liquid food supplements sound like an easy out, they may not always be the best choice. If you drink them in place of healthful eating, you will miss out on other naturally occurring nutrients, such as fiber and phytochemicals. So try adding dry milk powder to baked goods and casseroles, and buy yogurt and milk with added milk solids.

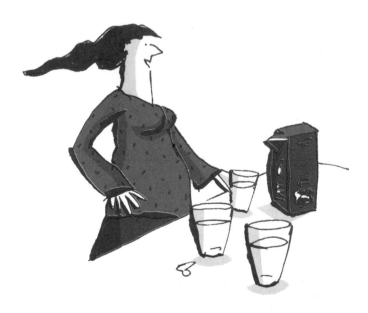

what to eat

twins: other protein foods

Some of the best foods to eat to boost your twins' protein intake
are cheese, brewer's yeast, pumpkin seeds, nuts and peanut butter
(unless you have a nut allergy or a family history of atopy),
seafood, beef and poultry, and soybean products. When planning
your snacks and meals, reach for foods that will help boost your
protein intake. For example, instead of a bowl of pretzels, grab a
handful of nuts; or put peanut butter on your toast instead of
regular butter. Add brewer's yeast to fruit smoothie drinks; sprinkle
cereals and casseroles with wheat germ; add nuts to cereal; toss
pumpkin seeds into salads; sprinkle shredded cheese into pasta;
add slices of low-fat cheese to sandwiches; and substitute one-
quarter soy flour for regular flour in baking.

As you can see, you can still eat a wide choice of protein-
enriched foods even if you don't like meat or eggs (and when
you're pregnant, you should eat only well-cooked eggs anyway,

not raw or undercooked ones). And perhaps you can find ways of hiding eggs in foods that you do like. For instance, crêpes contain eggs, yet they don't taste "eggy." Add eggs to ground turkey to make turkey burgers, or bake some egg custard. Rice pudding (*see page 161*) contains lots of eggs and milk, yet doesn't taste much like either.

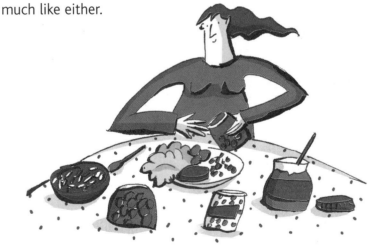

eat great on a budget

Not many of us have an unlimited grocery budget, but you don't have to sacrifice good nutrition just because you want to pinch your pennies. A container of whole oatmeal, for example, is much cheaper—and will last a lot longer—than a box of sugary cereal. Buy generic: you may be surprised, but the generic brand is often just as good as the prettier-packaged ones. In fact, most of the companies that make popular "brands" also make the generic versions. Sometimes, too, you can choose frozen over fresh—nutritionally, frozen concentrate juices and frozen veggies are just as valuable and sometimes cheaper. Frozen veggies are often even a bit more nutritious than their fresh counterparts, because they were frozen at the time of picking, rather than traveling on a truck for many days.

in season

Learn to eat in season and you'll not only save money but appreciate many fruits and vegetables more. Eating apples only in the fall is a great way to look forward to them each year, as is eating citrus fruit in the winter, asparagus in the spring, and soft fruit such as raspberries in the summer. Take advantage of the lower cost and the fact that all of these vegetables and fruits are at their nutritional best during their natural season.

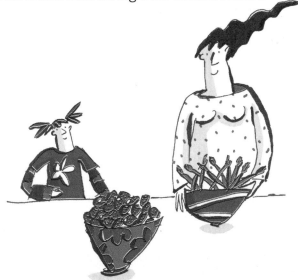

eating out

Of course, eating in is always the best way to ensure you know exactly what you are eating, but sometimes a girl just wants a night out! So choose the best restaurant available to you—one with a good salad bar, an option for fewer fried foods, and maybe even not-so-bad-for-you desserts. Turn your nonalcoholic drinking choice into a treat: most restaurants (particularly those with bars) have a variety of fruit juices available. If you're feeling a little left out, order your orange or grapefruit juice with some soda water and have them put it in a wineglass. And opt for whole grains: get your sandwich on a whole-grain bread, and take a second look at that bread basket. Most likely the rolls are made from bleached, processed white flour—not a great option at any time! If you eat out a lot, you might have to get used to skipping the bread altogether, or seek out a restaurant that prides itself on its bread selection.

what to eat

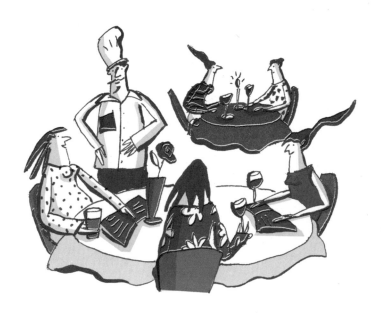

Ask questions: don't be afraid to "grill" the server (or even the chef). These days, they are used to getting questions about a variety of food issues, including allergens and the like—so don't be afraid to speak up and ask exactly what is in your food.

what to eat

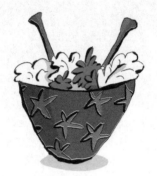

at work

It's hard to eat well at work, with vending machines just down the hall and a diner around the corner, but it can be done. I had a cabinet in my desk that became a virtual pantry for healthful snacks. Keep whole-grain crackers, a small jar of peanut butter, dried fruit, granola bars, and herbal teas or decaffeinated instant coffee. Get into the habit of using the office refrigerator and bring yogurts and other healthful foods to store there. And take some time, when you're not feeling ill, to pack your lunch bag. You can put tuna salad in a whole-grain pita and take some raw vegetables to munch on. Create a chef salad with dark greens, hard-cooked eggs, lean turkey, a bit of cheese—whatever you feel like.

stock up

Stock up on your favorite foods: buy larger quantities at one time and freeze them for later use. Buying something in bulk is always cheaper than buying a little at a time. You can also make meals ahead of time when you find a good deal—this will save you time as well as money.

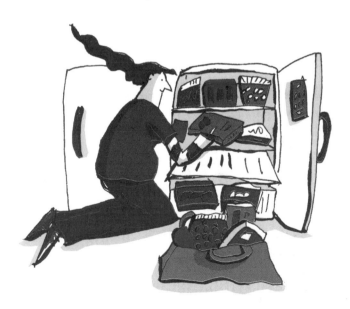

great tools

Here's the fun part of eating better: you can buy some new stuff! If you can't afford to buy brand new, then head to your local thrift store or dedicate a few Saturdays to yard sales, as most people rotate their kitchen items every so often and are always looking to get rid of the extras.

🖐 A steamer is a great item to have. You can buy an insert for an existing pot and steam your veggies into a healthful dinner.

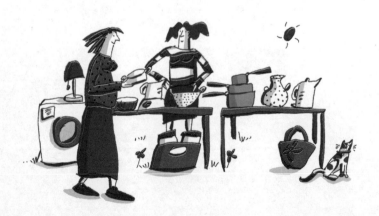

🖐 Look for nonstick skillets and bakeware, since they will eliminate your need to fry and bake with oil or butter.

🖐 Nylon, heat-resistant spatulas and spoons are essential to prevent damaging your new nonstick cookware.

🖐 A meat thermometer will help ensure that all of your meats are cooked through, eliminating potentially hazardous bacteria.

🖐 A small scale for weighing portions is helpful if you're keeping an eye on your weight gain.

🖐 Be sure to use a separate sponge for your dishes from the one you use for wiping counters. Once those sponges get "icky," either soak them in a solution of one capful of bleach to two cups of hot water for 15 minutes or so, or discard them and buy some new ones.

fish is really good for you

Besides tasting delicious and adding variety to your diet, fish
and seafood are highly nutritious, providing top-quality protein,
vitamins A, B (including B12), and D, important minerals (such as
iron, calcium, iodine, and phosphorus), and essential fatty acids
(such as omega-3). Research has shown that eating fish is an
excellent dietary habit to get into, and at no time is this more
important than during and after pregnancy. Fatty fish and fish
oils are among the richest sources of vitamins A and D, and the
age-old practice of giving children a spoonful of cod liver oil
each day to ward off winter chills and ills was highly effective.
However, because cod liver and halibut oils have such a high
vitamin A content, it's best not to take these supplements during
pregnancy unless they have been prescribed by your doctor,
and to eat fish in its natural state instead. However, the FDA
recommends that pregnant women should not eat shark,

swordfish, king mackerel, or tilefish, because of their high mercury content; tuna consumption should also be limited; and raw fish, sushi, and shellfish should be avoided during pregnancy.

Although fish is not as rich a source of calcium as milk and dairy products, research in South Africa has shown that women who eat whole canned fish (including the tiny bones in fish such as sardines) can obtain an appreciable amount of their daily calcium requirement from them. And fish is rich in phosphorus, which also helps strengthen your baby's bones and teeth and regulates the nervous system.

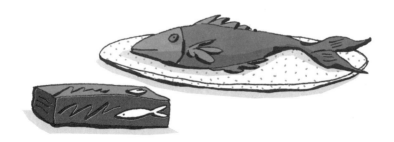

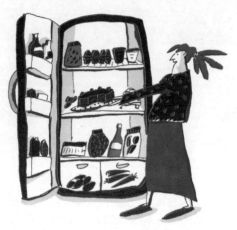

clean out the refrigerator

How do you get past those horrible reminders lurking in your
kitchen—the ones that remind you that you didn't always eat as
well as you've resolved to now? Clean out the cabinets, the
pantry, and the refrigerator! Do you have a stash of candy bars,
or a cupboard with too many cookies? Take them to work: the
folks there will love you, and you won't be tempted anymore.
Have half a cake lurking in the refrigerator? Freeze it: you'll have
just the right thing to serve when friends come over.

eat regular meals

Eating regular meals during pregnancy is one way of ensuring that you feel well and don't get the blues from low blood sugar. If you can't face breakfast right away during the first three months of pregnancy, when many moms-to-be are plagued by nausea, nibble a dry cracker or suck a slice of lemon or ice cubes when you wake to dispel the nausea. When you are feeling better, eat a light breakfast of fruit and cereal with yogurt. Dividing your food intake into six small meals a day is another good way to combat nausea, prevent bloating, and ensure a good nutrient intake. And having a glass of milk at night with a whole-wheat cookie can help you fall asleep, because milk is rich in tryptophan, an amino acid that promotes sleep. Or put two tablespoons of honey in a glass of buttermilk and stir in the juice of one lemon (good for those who are lactose intolerant [*see page 154*] or unable to drink plain milk without a belly rumble).

you're in it together

Eating correctly is not just good for the pregnant mom—it's good for the whole family . . . whether they believe you or not! If you are in charge of the family meals, then you are in a much better position to institute changes than a mom who isn't. If you bring home only whole-grain breads, leafy green veggies, and lean meats, then your family will have to eat them! Shop with your baby in mind and prepare meals that suit your newfound resolve to eat well (a few good recipes are given on *pages 156–163*). Your husband or partner—being the wonderful person they are—should understand this and be willing to participate in your efforts (just don't yell at them too much if you find a cookie bag in their car!). As for the kids—well, at this point you should pretty much have the "Eat what I put in front of you" ritual down pat. But whatever you do, don't "blame" the baby for the fact that there aren't any cookies in the pantry.

what to eat

Let them all know it's a lifestyle change—and not the baby's fault. Do your best to replace their familiar candies with sweet alternatives such as granola, oatmeal cookies, and other goodies. If this is your first baby, then following this way of eating now (and continuing after he or she is born) will ensure a child who isn't shocked by the brown bread in his lunch bag when he goes off to school.

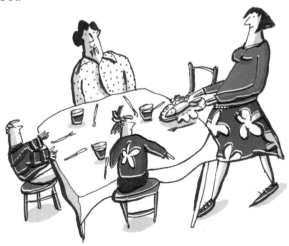

the effects of alcohol

Just one drink? Drinking alcohol during pregnancy is one of those things you need to discuss with your health-care provider. My advice? Just don't drink. And I'll tell you why: I've read so many studies that say all alcohol is bad, or some is bad, or one or two drinks a week is fine, that it's just impossible to tell. What *is* known is that too much alcohol can have a bad effect on your

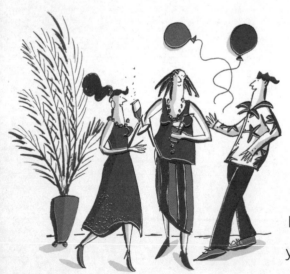

baby, whether by increasing your risk of miscarriage or, if you drink heavily, by causing fetal alcohol syndrome. It can be hard—particularly if you are a social drinker—to give it up, but just remember: "When the mother drinks, the baby drinks, too." For me, it was just easier not to drink at all. I've never been much of a drinker anyway, so it wasn't that difficult, but I never felt left out at parties. People always go out of their way to provide a nonalcoholic alternative for the preggie one. A couple of solutions, especially for social events, are to drink virgin daiquiris or Bloody Marys (in their virgin state, these are actually quite nutritious). Or, for those BYOB events, just take your own milk shake!

If you've discovered you are pregnant and suddenly recall that night you had a few too many (or maybe even a few of those nights), don't stress yourself out. It's unlikely that you harmed your baby, but do inform your health-care provider so that she can reassure you. Be honest with her about how much you drink: she isn't there to judge you, but to help you deliver a healthy baby.

kicking the caffeine habit

I'm not one to talk, because I get a headache without my morning coffee. But to give your baby the best odds of being born healthy, it's a good idea to cut down on caffeine (the FDA recommends having less than three cups of coffee a day)—if not quit altogether. Research has shown that mothers who drink strong coffee have smaller babies than those who don't. Lack of caffeine can make you tired and cranky, so try to find other "lifts" in your day. My favorite lift was a couple of cookies in the afternoon—although a more appropriate lift would be exercise or a high-protein snack! Remember that Ceylon tea, cola drinks, and sodas also contain caffeine. I found that mixing seltzer with juice was a great alternative.

herbal iced tea

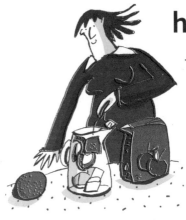

There are plenty of other nutritious drinks for expectant moms, without having to load your unborn baby with excessive caffeine. I made a lot of herbal iced tea.

ingredients

For a pitcher of tea, you need: 2 pt (1.2 l) boiling water; 5–6 herbal tea bags (I liked raspberry zinger); juice and zest of 3–4 oranges or lemons; ice cubes; sugar to taste

Put the herbal tea bags into a pitcher with the water and steep for 15 minutes. Add the citrus juice and zest, then fill up the pitcher with ice cubes and add sugar (not aspartame!) to taste.

water, water everywhere

Drinking plenty of liquids—especially pure water—is an excellent way of helping your body flush out waste products through the skin, kidneys, and bowels. Remember that you are doing double cleansing duty while you are pregnant. You will be doing yourself and your baby a good turn if you have a high intake of liquids, but avoid gassy cold drinks (especially artificially sweetened ones), which can make you feel nauseated. And until more research has been done on the possible effect of artificial sweeteners on fetal development, it's a good idea to avoid these products altogether during pregnancy.

If you live in areas where the water is suspect, boil any water that you intend to drink, and cool it before using it. Water filters are also a possibility—and there are less expensive versions these days. Aim to drink six glasses of water every day, and make a point of having fruit juices (the sort you squeeze yourself will be the freshest of all, and will give you a virtuous buzz), red bush tea, and milk to supplement your liquid intake. Just remember that bought orange juice should contain "100% orange juice" (from actual, grown-on-a-tree oranges)—not "100% orange flavor."

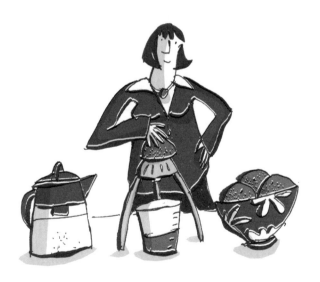

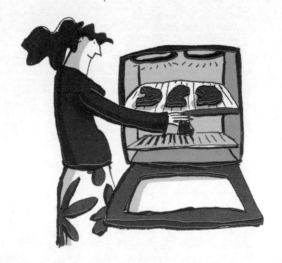

low fat doesn't mean low taste

Here are some simple ideas to help you eliminate excess fat from your diet, if you're trying to stop your weight gain from running away with you. I, for one, am in love with butter and olive oil, but I found that by following some of these easy tips from other moms, I could still spread the butter on a (whole-grain) bagel in the morning.

what to eat

🖐 Cook in a nonstick pan, and use water or stock to keep your food from sticking.

🖐 Grill meats instead of frying them—the fat drips off, instead of swamping your food.

🖐 Roast meats on a raised rack in your roasting pan, so that the juices drip into the pan.

🖐 Substitute applesauce for half of the oil in a cake recipe. I've done this many times and no one could ever tell the difference!

🖐 Reduce the fat in salad dressing by replacing half of the oil with water. For creamy dressings, use buttermilk, yogurt, or cottage cheese instead of sour cream or mayonnaise.

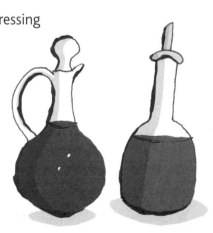

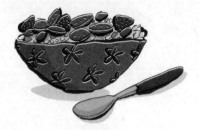

sugar, sugar, sugar

Don't ban sugar altogether: some sugar, added to wholesome
foods, may make them more appetizing—for instance, a little
brown sugar on oatmeal. The sugar listed on food labels is often
a combination of naturally occurring sugar and added sugar. If
you spot the ending "-ose," it is sugar in disguise! Other sugar-
in-hiding includes syrup, honey, corn sweetener, corn syrup, fruit-
juice concentrate, high-fructose corn syrup, and invert sugar.
Reduce the amount of sugar in baking: you can often lose up to
one-third with no detectable change in the end product. Bagels,
whole-grain muffins, or tortillas can replace doughnuts or cakes.
And top cereal with fresh fruit, which adds natural sweetness.

desserts

Don't make desserts a regular part of every meal—save them for special treats, but do enjoy them on the weekend or on family occasions. Serve fresh fruit for dessert on weekdays. You'll be getting an extra-healthful food, without ignoring your sweet tooth. Also use fresh fruit to sweeten plain yogurt: puréed berries mixed with yogurt makes a great snack to have midafternoon.

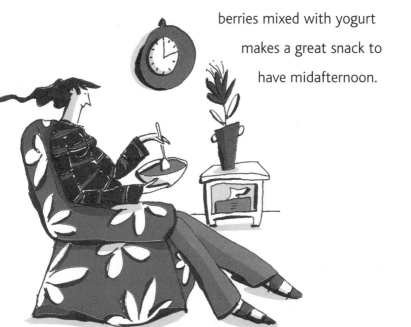

baby teeth

Many women have heard that calcium from a mother's teeth can be lost during pregnancy—and have even asked me about it. Dentist Kim Loos says, "There is no scientific data to suggest that calcium is lost from a mother's teeth during pregnancy. I am not sure how this falsehood originated, but it has been perpetuated so often that many people incorrectly accept it as fact. The calcium your baby requires is provided by eating a balanced diet, not by your teeth."

Pregnant women need 1,000 mg of calcium per day to maintain their own teeth and bones and help build their child's. At least three servings of milk, cheese, or yogurt each day should provide adequate calcium. However, if you *do* become deficient in dietary calcium, your obstetrician may recommend supplements to ensure that your bones do not lose calcium and become weakened, leading to a risk of osteoporosis later on.

what to eat

Make sure that you don't neglect your teeth during pregnancy. Hormonal changes alter the oral environment and render your teeth more susceptible to decay. Many moms-to-be increase snacking during pregnancy, and although this is quite normal, the frequency of snacking inevitably influences tooth decay. So be sure that you brush and floss your teeth carefully after every meal and snack.

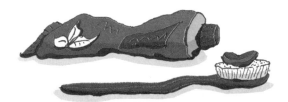

what to eat

lactose intolerance

During pregnancy, you may experience symptoms that are
interpreted as lactose intolerance, although it's rare for a true
intolerance to develop as a result of pregnancy. What may work
for you now is reducing the amount of dairy foods that you eat
at one time. For example, instead of a whole glass of milk, have
just a half glass. Eat and drink smaller amounts—but do so more
frequently. Some dairy products are better tolerated than others
in pregnancy. For instance, yogurt (whose lactose is already
partially digested by the cultured bacteria) may be easier to
digest, whereas fat will take longer. Choose low-
fat or nonfat cheeses and dairy products
and skim milk. If the symptoms
continue, try drinking lactose-reduced
milk or taking Lactaid tablets, to see if
that eases the situation.

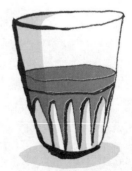

what to eat

a reading lesson

Sure, the labels may say they're wholesome foods, but are they?
Your new eating habits mean you will have to become one of
those women you see in the supermarket who read all the
labels. I know, I know . . . but get used to it! You'll be shocked to
find out how many "wholesome" breads contain bleached flour
or high-fructose corn syrup. Never fall for words like "all-natural,"
"light," or "organic" unless the ingredients list can prove it.

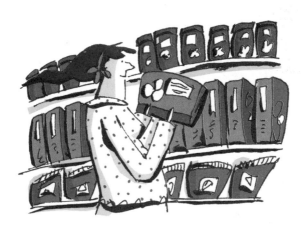

bean and pasta soup

This is a dish that has everything: protein, carbohydrates, vitamins, and minerals—a great meal that nourishes both soul and body.

ingredients

For 8 servings, you need: 2 cups beans (a 1 lb/450 g bag) of your choice (a mixed soup blend is colorful); water to cover (2–2½ quarts/ 1.2–1.5 l); 2½ quarts (1.2–1.5 l) stock (chicken, beef, or vegetable); 1 large onion, chopped (about 2 cups); 1–2 cups grated carrots; 1–2 cups chopped celery; 3 or 4 cloves garlic, minced (optional); 1 lb (450 g) plum (or other) tomatoes, skinned and chopped (or use a 14 oz/400 g can); 1 tbsp fresh basil (or 1 tsp dried), or a little oregano, marjoram, savory, etc. (whatever herb smells and/or tastes good to you); 1 tbsp fresh parsley, chopped (or 1 tsp dried); 1 cup pasta of your choice, small or broken into pieces; 1 lb (450 g) sausage (sweet, hot, or a combination), cooked, drained of fat, and crumbled

what to eat

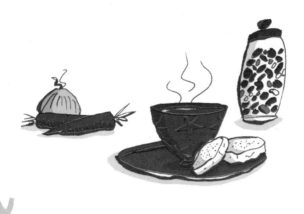

The night before you want to serve your soup, cover the beans with water. Let them soak until about 1½–2 hours before your meal. Drain them and place in a soup pot, then add the stock. Stir in all the other ingredients except the pasta and sausage, then bring to a boil and let simmer until the beans are almost tender.

Add the pasta and sausage, then simmer the soup until the pasta is just tender. Serve the soup accompanied by a green salad and a loaf of crusty bread.

roasted veggie pizza

Have your pizza and eat it, too! This
crust is ungreasy, bready, and wonderful,
and you can vary the toppings.

ingredients

For 1 medium-crust 18 x 13-inch (45 x 33-cm) pizza, or 2 thin-crust,
12-inch (30-cm) round pizzas, you need:

Crust: 2¾ cups unbleached all-purpose flour; ½ cup semolina flour
or coarse cornmeal; 1¼ tsp salt; 2 tsp sugar; 2 tbsp olive oil; 1 tsp
instant yeast; 1 cup plus 2 tbsp water

Filling: 1 cup (8 oz/225 g) ricotta cheese; ⅓ cup prepared pesto sauce;
½ cup Parmesan cheese, grated; salt and pepper to taste

Topping: a variety of sliced vegetables roasted until cooked, but not
quite brown (25–30 minutes) in a preheated oven at 425°F (220°C)

Mix together all of the crust ingredients and knead (by hand, mixer, bread machine, or food processor) until you have a soft, smooth dough. Place in a lightly greased bowl, then cover and let rise for 1 hour. Gently deflate the dough and put it back in the bowl, then cover and refrigerate for several hours or overnight.

To make the filling, combine the ricotta, pesto, Parmesan, and salt and pepper in a small bowl. Refrigerate until ready to use.

To assemble the pizza, divide the dough into two pieces or leave in one piece (for a thicker crust). Roll or pat into the desired thickness and shape. Place on a lightly greased pan, then cover and let rest for 30 minutes while you preheat your oven to 400°F (200°C). To cook, bake the pizza dough for 10 minutes. Remove, deflate any bubbles, and spread with the filling, then layer on the roasted vegetables. Return to the oven and bake for another 12–15 minutes, or until the cheese is bubbly and the crust is golden brown.

succulent salmon fillets

Salmon cooks beautifully in the
microwave and is full of goodness. These
fillets have little need of embellishment.

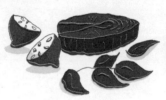

ingredients

For 2 servings, you need: 2 pieces of 6-oz (175-g) salmon fillets; salt
and freshly ground pepper; juice of ½ lemon (optional); a sprinkling of
fresh chopped herbs, such as basil, dill, or tarragon (optional)

Rinse the fillets and pat dry, then place them on a microwave-safe plate.
Season and sprinkle with lemon juice and herbs, if desired. Cover the
dish tightly with plastic wrap, piercing it a few times. Microwave for
2–3 minutes, or until the fish is opaque. Stand for 1–2 minutes, then
check to see if the salmon is done. Return to the microwave for another
½–1 minute if necessary. Pour the cooking juices over the fish and serve.

sweet rice and raisin pudding

Try this perennial favorite for breakfast, dessert, or a snack. One serving provides 150 mg of calcium, plus lots of high-quality protein and plenty of B vitamins.

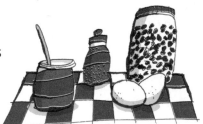

ingredients

For 2 servings, you need: 2 cups cooked brown rice; 2 eggs; 2 cups milk; ¼ cup nonfat dry milk powder; ½ tsp cinnamon; ½ cup raisins; ½ tsp vanilla; ⅓ cup honey

Preheat the oven to 350°F (180°C). Combine all the ingredients, then pour them into a greased baking dish. Sprinkle with freshly grated nutmeg and bake for 30 minutes, or until set. Serve hot, warm, or cold.

cranberry apricot bread

This quick bread (a great source of vitamin C) features dried
cranberries, apricots, and nuts nestling in an orange- and

cinnamon-scented batter. If you're planning
on serving a turkey during the holidays,
this bread makes a great accompaniment.

ingredients

For 1 loaf (about 16 servings), you need: ½ cup butter (at room
temperature); ¾ cup sugar; ¼ tsp orange oil or 2 tsp orange zest,
grated; ½ tsp salt; 1 tsp baking powder; 1 tsp cinnamon; ½ tsp
nutmeg; 3 eggs; 1¾ cups unbleached all-purpose flour; ½ cup milk;
1 cup dried cranberries; ½ cup dried apricots, diced or slivered;
½ cup pecans or walnuts, chopped (optional)

what to eat

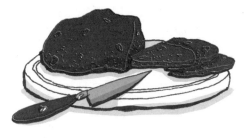

Preheat the oven to 350°F (180°C). Using a medium-size mixing bowl, cream together the butter, sugar, orange oil or zest, salt, baking powder, and spices until well blended. Beat in the eggs one at a time, whisking until fluffy after each addition. Stir in the flour, then add half the milk at a time, mixing well after each addition. Gently stir in the cranberries, apricots, and nuts.

Spoon the batter into a lightly greased 8½ x 4½-inch (22 x 12-cm) loaf pan. Bake the bread for 50–55 minutes, or until a skewer inserted in the center comes out clean. Remove the bread from the oven, and let it cool in the pan for 10 minutes. Turn the loaf out and let it cool completely on a wire rack.

what to wear

"Wahhh! I don't look pregnant—I just look frumpy!"
This is a common frustration early in the second trimester.
In fact, 63 percent of moms polled around their 15th week
of pregnancy claimed to be experiencing this unpleasant
transitional stage. Your belly may be blooming just enough
to make your regular clothes uncomfortable, but at the
same time maternity clothes are simply huge.

Thank heaven those "Baby on the Way" T-shirts are
a thing of the past—as are those floral muu-muus! Today
even the world's top designers have maternity lines and
there are more clothing options available to you than ever
before. I hated shopping for maternity clothes (mostly

what to wear

because with each child, I didn't consider the possibility of the next one), and I didn't want to spend money on items that I'd wear just for a few months. So here are some tips to help you find what you need, save money while you do so, and make use of whatever you (or your partner) already has in the clothes closet.

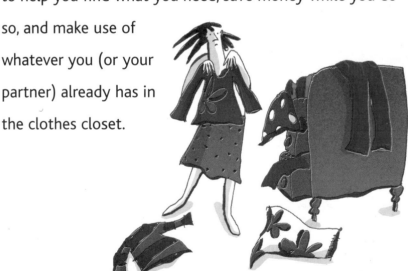

value for money

The prohibitive element of buying maternity clothes continues to be the monetary investment for clothing that gets worn for such a short length of time. But there are solutions to this problem.

☙ Get the most out of your purchases: There are clothes you can buy that will take you all the way from pregnancy to nursing. There are also inexpensive matching sets that can be purchased, and when you add a few colored T-shirts, these give you a whole attractive wardrobe for a lot less than you'd spend on two really nice outfits.

☙ Beg, borrow, and steal: Ask friends or relatives if they have clothing you can borrow, since clothes often get passed around circles of pregnant friends.

☙ Wear them big: Plus-size clothing can lessen the cost of the items you are buying, although they will not fit as well as clothes made specifically for pregnancy.

what to wear

🖐 Raid your husband's closet: If your mate is larger than you, feel free to help yourself to his clothing; tell him I told you to . . .

🖐 Discounts: Shop at yard sales, discount outlets, consignment shops, or end-of-year sales. I found out about my first pregnancy in March and raided the winter closeouts for my December due date. I saved a lot of money and got some nice clothes to wear.

🖐 Make your own! If you're even slightly handy with sewing, making your own clothes should be fairly easy to do.

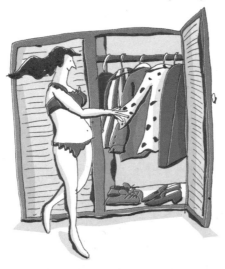

don't scrimp on the basics

Invest in a good bra. Whether you're planning a night on the town or an afternoon lounging around the house, you'll look and feel better if your underwear is comfortable. Your breasts will swell during pregnancy—some women go up by as much as three cup sizes—so look for bras made of 100 percent cotton with wide straps and bands to support growing breast tissue.

A good maternity bra should have several rows of adjustable hooks in back to accommodate expansion. Most specialty stores and large department stores stock maternity bras, panties, panty hose, and slips.

Get professionally fitted for a bra: it's free, so it's worth it.

My first pregnancy, I shelled out big bucks for some fancy (but actually rather plain) maternity bikini underwear, but by the end of pregnancy I had abandoned them for some delightful granny-style panties. With my third pregnancy, I found that the regular bikini underwear that I bought in a size larger than normal really worked best, although occasionally nothing felt as good as my granny underwear!

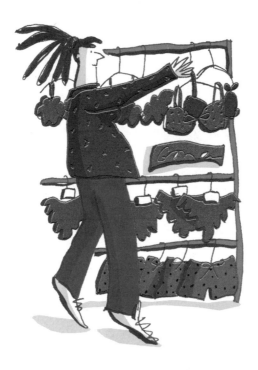

what to wear

if you're tall . . .

☀ Knee-length skirts look great on you, because they help to break up the length of your body.

☀ Don't dress all in one color—it will make you look even taller. Instead, mix and match colors.

☀ Experiment with horizontal stripes and patterns, which will work well on your tall frame.

☀ Try long jackets, either worn with pants or over a dress.

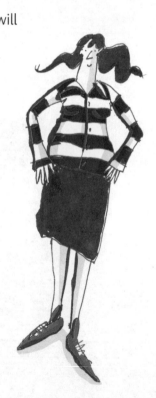

if you're petite . . .

 Stick with monochromatic tops and bottoms, which will lengthen your body. It helps if shoes and stockings match, too.

 Go with slim-fitting styles instead of bulky ones—they won't overwhelm your delicate frame.

 If you're curvy on the bottom, remember: dark colors are slimming, so choose pants, skirts, and dresses in the classic hues of black, brown, navy, dark gray, and wine.

 Stock up on boat-neck and other high-neck tops, which draw the eye upward. A choker, short strand of pearls, or a scarf will also work well.

 Avoid horizontal stripes, which will make you look wider than you are.

 Try menswear-style shirts—they will minimize your hips.

find a flattering swimsuit

Take pride in your pregnant body, and find a swimsuit that flatters you and feels comfortable, no matter what your body type; swimming is great exercise and this is one clothing investment that's worth it.

✋ Short legs: Wear a suit with higher-cut leg openings. Your legs will look longer because this cut creates the illusion of length.

✋ Large hips: To minimize your hips, wear a suit with low-cut leg openings, which offer the most hip coverage. Go for a solid, dark color for the bottom half of your suit. Or look for a stripe or design along the bust area to draw the eye upward. Alternately, try a suit with a short skirt to minimize your hip area.

✋ Large bust: If pregnancy has increased your bust size so much that you feel self-conscious, you can flatter it with a suit that has a high neck and a supportive shelf or cup bra. A dark-colored top and a light-colored bottom will further minimize it.

what to wear

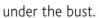 Small bust: If you want to create cleavage, wear a suit with a V-neck and underwire support, or a halter-style top that lifts the bust. To generally enhance your bustline, wear a suit with a ruffle, texture, or stripes along the bust. Avoid high-neck suits because these tend to press breasts down.

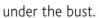 Bold patterns: Generally, avoid these if you're pregnant. Instead go for smaller prints, colorful piping, and horizontal stripes along or under the bust.

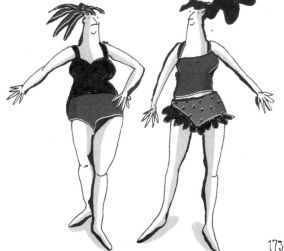

mix 'n' match

Buy pieces of clothing that mix and match with each other. Look for clothes that are not necessarily sold in maternity departments, such as tunics; oversize sweaters, sweatshirts and blouses; loose-fitting dresses; and knit stirrup pants. You may even be able to wear some of these items after the baby is born. Choose fabrics that span the seasons: cotton, wool gabardine, denim, challis, khaki, rayon, or easy-care polyester blends. For a psychological boost, spread out your purchases over the pregnancy, so you have something new every couple of months.

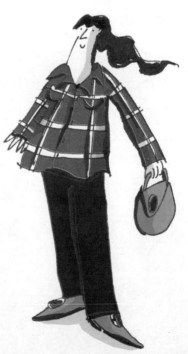

what should you buy?

The kind of maternity clothing you buy depends on when you are pregnant and on your budget, as well as your lifestyle. But you can create a "capsule wardrobe" easily and inexpensively by buying a pack of oversize T-shirts in different colors, a couple of solid-color skirts or pants (with elastic waistbands), and comfortable leggings. These three components can be combined to see you through work, outings, and time spent at home. Couple them with your favorite accessories, and you have a look that can take you almost anywhere.

what to wear

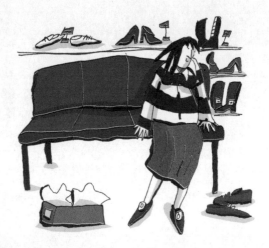

treat your feet right

This means choosing shoes that are roomy and comfortable and that offer adequate support. According to the American College of Foot and Ankle Surgeons, your feet may grow permanently by a half to a full size during pregnancy. ACFAS recommends wearing an arch support to help sustain the extra weight your feet will be carrying; wearing athletic shoes with a roomy toe box; and support stockings to minimize foot and ankle swelling.

keep in mind . . .

Keep one thing in mind when planning your maternity wardrobe. Maternity sizing is a guess. It is not only relative to your pre-pregnancy size, but is also affected by the number of babies you are carrying, how you carry them, and the amount of weight that you gain. You won't know the last two variables until after the need for maternity clothing arises. So, if you are a normal medium who sees a bargain of (or gets an offer to borrow) a maternity small—take it. You can get lots of wear out of the item, even if it won't fit at the very end of your term.

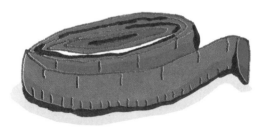

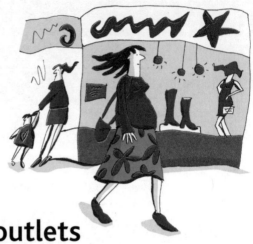

maternity outlets

Try a maternity outlet store if you need clothes to wear to the office. This is where I blew the bulk of my maternity budget, almost entirely on work clothes. The chain I went to, Maternity Works, has branches in outlet malls around the country and sells clothes from a range of boutiques. All outlet stores tend to have a mix of real bargains and almost-full-priced merchandise, so once you're there you need to do some careful hunting through the clothes racks to find those genuine discounts.

check out sales racks

You know those loose-fitting dresses that those in the fashion world try to foist on us every few years? The ones that you look at and say; "Yeah, right, everyone will think I'm pregnant if I wear this." Well, you're not the only one. These styles seem to end up on sales racks or in outlet stores at the end of the season. When you're pregnant, though, wearing something that looks like a maternity dress is a fine idea. I got two dresses for work this way.

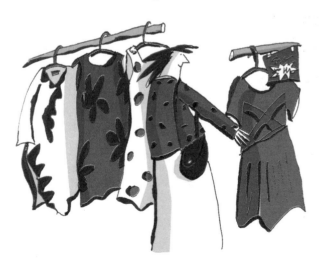

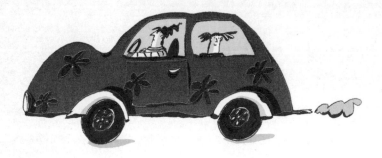

belt up

You have a responsibility for your baby's safety as well as your own, so make it a habit to securely buckle your seat belt every time you travel by car. The shoulder and lap-belt combination is recommended. Position the lap belt low across your hips, below your expanding abdomen, and the shoulder portion across your chest and abdomen. In an accident, the seat belt will prevent you and your unborn child from crashing into the dashboard or being thrown from the car. If you are in an accident, contact your health-care provider for advice, even if you don't appear to be injured.

layer your clothing

Your metabolic rate increases by about 20 percent when you're pregnant, which means that if everyone else is shivering, you're just as likely to be complaining about the heat. With a layered look, you can peel clothes off as needed. On cold days, put a T-shirt or polo under a sweater, or wear a turtleneck under a vest.

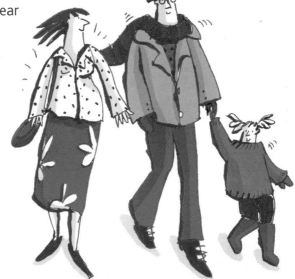

support yourself

Don't wear restrictive clothing such as tight belts and girdles, or socks or stockings with elastic bands. Do wear maternity support panty hose or stockings, available at most maternity clothing stores. You don't want anything restrictive around your mid-section, but you do want to keep the blood flowing, which is the reason for support stockings. Pull them on before getting out of bed in the morning and before the blood has a chance to pool in your legs, to help minimize the risk of varicose veins. They can also help prevent circulation problems in a car or on a plane.

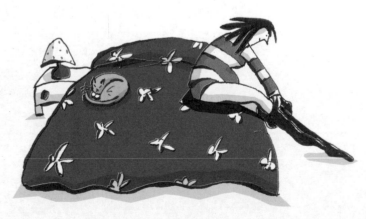

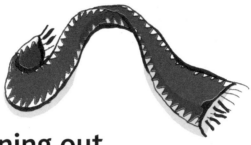

an evening out

"I'm 33 weeks," one mom said, "but not overly huge. I have a long, formal full skirt, the type that you wear with a matching sweater set or silk top. Well, I wore this, but just didn't zip it all the way. Then I had a nice long black sweater that I just wore with it. It worked very well, and everyone commented that they couldn't believe how fashionable maternity dress outfits were."

I found a simple black maternity dress best for me, but if that doesn't work, try a sweater and long black skirt. You can add elegance with something sparkly for the evening. Remember: accessories are a pregnant woman's best friend! Just adding a bright scarf to a black dress can make a big difference.

back to basics

"Early in my pregnancy," another mom said, "I splurged on a great loose-cut black jacket, the kind I could wear with jeans or a skirt. It wasn't a maternity jacket, but it took me through my whole pregnancy and I sometimes still wear it now. I'd say, spend the money on some basic item you love, because if you have to wear it a lot, you might as well enjoy it!"

She also found that shopping for plus-size cotton-knit stretch pants was far cheaper than buying actual maternity pants.

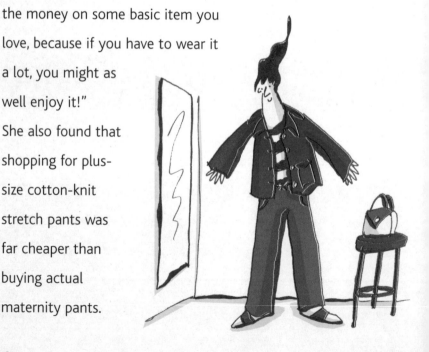

what to wear

splurge (a little)

Even if your budget doesn't allow for
a completely new wardrobe, invest
in one outfit that makes you feel
special. A sexy dress, black velvet
pants and a swingy top, or a stunning

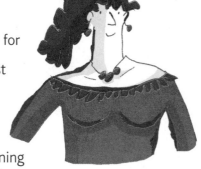

suit can make you look like a million dollars when you feel
anything but. A bootleg jumpsuit, a fabulous print dress, or a
coordinating pant suit will add a big splash of fashion to your
maternity wardrobe with minimal financial impact. Wear it as
much as possible, while you can. And accentuate the positive:

🖐 Gorgeous gams? Flaunt them in a short dress.

🖐 Upper arms to die for? Show them off with a sleeveless shirt.

🖐 Proud of your new, more expansive décolletage? Try a
revealing, low-cut top. You don't have to go undercover just
because you're pregnant.

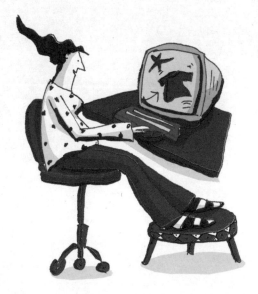

let your fingers do the typing

Shop online! You can shop at extensive online collections from a variety of maternity fashion outlets. Get what you like at the best prices, and save your aching back, your aching feet, your aching pubic bone, and so on, in the process. A good starting point is www.onlineclothingstores.com/Maternity.htm, which has links to a range of maternity clothing stores.

go classic

Certain clothes go a long way toward helping you feel "normal" during your pregnancy. Top maternity jeans with an oversize sweatshirt that you can also wear post-pregnancy and you won't feel quite as conspicuous in a crowd (for those of you who don't wish to be conspicuous, of course!). Also, if this is your first pregnancy, buy the best clothes you can afford, but don't buy trendy outfits—two or three years down the road, when you need to dig out those maternity clothes again, you may not believe you actually wore (or could fit into) those clothes. Make sure that you pick classic styles in plain, easy-to-match colors such as navy, cream, or tan, and—for winter—black (which is very slimming).

the power of makeup

"Makeup can do wonders for you during your pregnancy. It can be used as a tool to make you feel pretty and in control," says famed makeup artist Bobbi Brown. That's particularly important at this time when so many women feel they've lost control of their body. "Makeup can be washed off—it isn't permanent,"

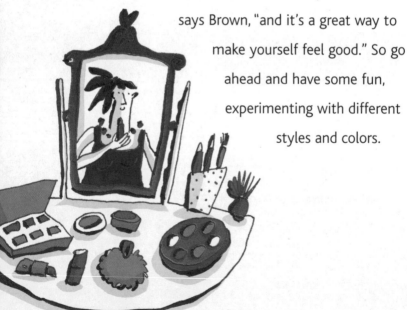

says Brown, "and it's a great way to make yourself feel good." So go ahead and have some fun, experimenting with different styles and colors.

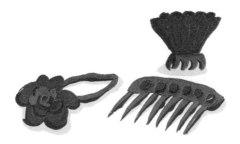

avoid hair-raising hairstyles

During pregnancy your hair goes into a growth phase—good news for some women, who find they now have shinier, thicker hair. But if you normally have a thick head of hair anyway, you may find a short cut easier to wear. "You don't have to go through a dramatic change," says Amina Rubio, stylist and colorist at the David Oliver Studio, a San Francisco hair salon. "Women get overwhelmed by the results when they do." Work with your stylist to find a cut that suits you. Rubio, a hair accessories designer, recommends using clips, barrettes, and combs to enhance your style. But don't overdo it. "Less is more," he says.

hone your fashion sense

Just because you're expecting, that doesn't mean you're relegated to wearing pastel clothing festooned with bows and lace. Gone are the days when a pregnant woman could dress only like a meringue. Black—the color of choice for chic, non-pregnant fashionistas—works wonders for future mommies as well. Jeans made for pregnant women are comfortable and are required wearing for feeling fashionable. There are many stretch jeans available for the pregnant mom: some have elastic fronts, others spandex ones; most also have features to help support your back. I loved the spandex fronts, but all moms have their preferences.

don't forget your skin

The same pregnancy hormones that put your emotions in an uproar can wreak havoc on your skin. Your complexion may look great, with that much-touted "pregnancy glow," or it may become drier than usual and splotchy. A good moisturizer can work wonders on your expanding belly—or anywhere your skin feels dry. And who knows? It may even diminish stretch marks. Although experts say moisturizers don't work, moms who've come through pregnancy stretch-mark free often swear by them.

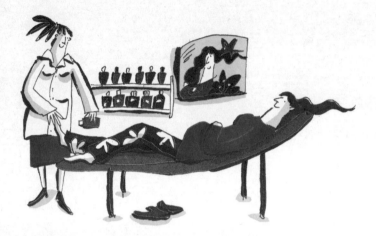

indulge in "the cures"

There's nothing like a manicure or pedicure ("mani-pedi" if you go for both) to lift the spirits and give your self-esteem a quick boost. What could be nicer than having a professional pamper your hands and feet while you relax and let someone else do the work for a change? And you could throw in a pregnancy massage for good measure: it's great to have someone else make you feel like a queen for a day.

flaunt that tummy

"My girlfriend Lori wore the slinkiest, tightest, silkiest clothes ever while she was pregnant, even letting her belly show under short tops a lot of the time (yes, it was summer)," says Karen Salmansohn in *Hot Mama: How to Have a Babe and Be a Babe*. "And she looked divine. There's nothing sexier than a pregnant woman who boldly and enthusiastically shows off her belly." If you have the confidence, flaunt that tummy.

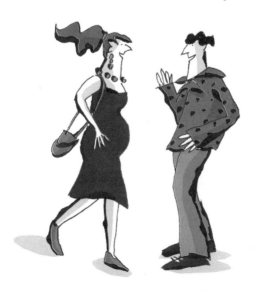

choosing shoes

For the traveling mom-to-be, nothing is more important than choosing comfortable, supportive footwear. The best shoes or sandals have a contoured foot bed to help prevent aches, and a thick, skid-resistant sole for good traction and support when walking. Sneakers built for high-impact aerobic sports fit the bill; strappy high heels and mules do not. Elastic inserts, ties, or adjustable straps are must-haves for when your feet swell. Here are some questions to ask yourself while shoe shopping:

🖐 Does it have a square toe? Not only are square toes in style, but the extra room helps ward off painful corns and bunions.

🖐 Does it have a broad, low heel? A simple loafer with a low, stacked heel offers much better support for your growing weight than a low-heeled pump.

🖐 Does it offer ankle support? Flat shoes are often better than heels, but some ballet flats and moccasins don't offer adequate ankle support. Walk around the store—if your foot lifts out of it, there's not enough support.

🖐 If it's an everyday shoe, does it have a rubber sole? These shock absorbers are easier on your knees and back. One great trend for pregnant women is "mock sneaks," which are athletic-style, slip-on, rubber-soled shoes in leather and suede.

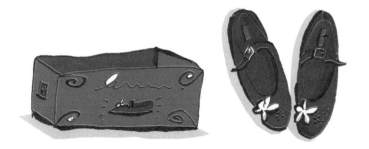

pre-pregnancy sizing

When shopping, start by selecting your pre-pregnancy size.
After all, your arms and legs don't get longer, and your basic
body structure will remain the same. Well-made maternity
clothes give you the extra room only where you need it—belly,
bust, hips, and arm holes—while maintaining the pre-pregnancy
proportions of each size range. "Front hemlines on tops and
jackets may be slightly longer earlier in your term to allow
for gradual leveling out as your belly expands," explain Teresa
Gallagher and Maria Mueller of Anna Cris Maternity. "Earlier on,
expect a little extra material in dresses and jackets to allow for
expansion: jacket clips or built-in ties are used to gather it back
until you need it"—and you will!

what to wear

choose easy-care fabrics

You are a walking hormone. You don't need hassles . . . So stick with soft, breathable clothing that is wash-and-wear. Do you need to be ironing? No. So check care directions religiously before you buy. You'll probably find yourself cycling through your maternity wardrobe faster than you would your regular one, so durable fabrics that can bear frequent washing are a big plus.

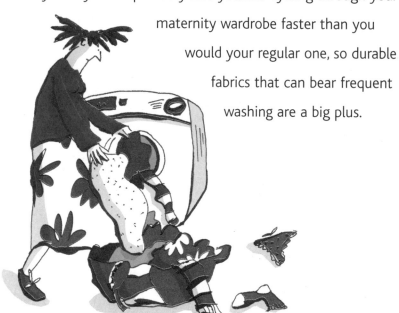

don't delay!

Why frustrate yourself by trying to expand waistlines with elastic bands and open buttons? With the exception of a very few people, buying maternity jeans will be inevitable, so don't delay. The more wear you are able to get out of your maternity clothes, the better your investment will be. So as soon as you can't zip up your favorite pair of jeans, treat yourself to the comfort of maternity jeans; topped with your everyday button-down white oxford, no one else will know the difference—but you will certainly feel it.

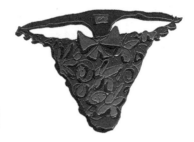

thongbird

All kinds of maternity undies are out there—from under-the-belly bikinis to up-to-the chest briefs. But did you know that maternity thongs are also available? Some women swear they're super-comfortable; others wear them simply because they make them feel like their old sexy selves. You might not want to wear them every day, though. Some doctors say they're seeing more thong-wearers complaining of vaginal infections, because bacteria is more able to travel from the rectum to the vagina. And hemorrhoid sufferers beware: thongs may irritate that sensitive tissue. Not worried? Then go ahead and relish the pantyline-free look!

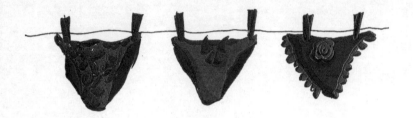

more on underwear

Sure, you want to look good, but don't you want to *feel* good, too? Of course you do. For our pregnant selves, comfort is of paramount importance. In that spirit, here is my best advice: go for bikini briefs and low-rise pants. I remember going to work wearing maternity undies, a slip, and a skirt—*three* waistbands! That's for the birds. By my second pregnancy, I learned that not only will nonmaternity panties work just fine, but they are often more comfortable. Get the claustrophobic waistbands away from my tummy! And let's just hope low-rise pants never go out of fashion for the maternity set.

talk yourself into a good mood

If all else fails, tell yourself that, even though you can't squeeze

into a pair of size-6 slacks right now, you're still fabulous.

Beauty is a state of grace, not a certain look, size, or weight.

You're glowing, you're pregnant, and you're beautiful. (And if

this doesn't work, you can always cover up all the mirrors in

your house, settle into a good book, and call it a day.)

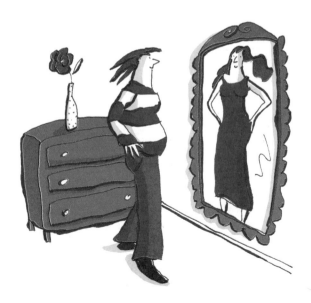

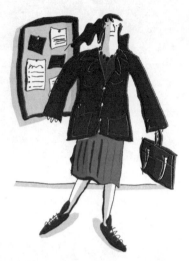

bigger isn't always better

When you see the prices on office-appropriate maternity wear, you may be tempted simply to shop for the next size up from your regular clothes. This strategy often works with casualwear, which is intended to fit loosely. However, if you use this tactic with office clothing, you'll end up with shoulders that are way too big, sleeves that are too long, and an overall look that can only be described as sloppy (at best).

stick with your style

That elusive quality known as "style" is something most of us don't think about too often, as we rush to get dressed without considering why we choose to dress in a certain fashion. But, as Cherie Serota and Jody Kozlow Gardner note in *Pregnancy Chic: The Fashion Survival Guide*, "The main point that we stress day in and day out is, at all costs hold on to your style. Maintain it during your pregnancy. Your style before you became pregnant should continue to be your style during your pregnancy. You are still the same person. Why should your whole sense of style change just because the EPT stick turned blue?" So keep to what you know really works for you.

focus on: detail and fabric

Fashion-conscious women ask all the time, "How can I maintain a sense of style when my body seems to have other plans for me?" If you think pregnancy is a nine-month sentence of overalls and leggings, take heart from the following tips.

🖐 Have an eye for detail: when you can't control the size you're wearing, you can at least select clothes with wonderful detailing—ruffled hems, notch necklines, cuffs, collars, fringes.

🖐 Focus on fabrics and textures: goodbye, plain cotton, hello to a new wave of fabulous-looking (and -feeling) fabrics, such as stretch denims, mesh prints, comfy knits, faux suedes, washable twills, and many more.

focus on: tops or bottoms

Start slowly and work your way up, selecting clothes that will
work well together. For your first pieces, try to stick with basics
that will go with everything. Black leggings, denim jeans, twill
pants, and a short cotton interlock skirt are a few ideas for basic

bottoms that
allow creative
combinations with
any color or print top.
Or, if you prefer to
wear your tops as your
basics, try a white or
classic French blue button-
down oxford, a denim
shirt, or a solid color
cotton/spandex tunic top.

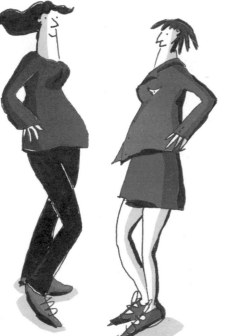

back to the future

Plan on a little post-pregnancy shopping. New mothers shouldn't feel too pressured to fit into their old jeans right after the baby is born. Instead, plan to buy a couple of new transition pieces that will last until you get your pre-pregnancy shape back. Think ahead to what you'll need after maternity leave. Your shape at three to four months may correspond to the size you'll be when you return to work. Select clothes to fit you in early pregnancy that will be appropriate, season-wise, for your return.

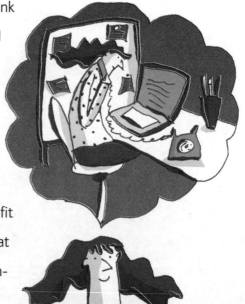

gently does it

Take a wait-and-see attitude when purchasing work clothes, say Teresa Gallagher and Maria Mueller. "If you need a two-piece suit, start with one great style that makes you feel every bit as professional as you did before. If you need black or dark blue, look for some texture in the material, such as a ribbing, to add some interest."

Try to fit your basic wardrobe into your work wardrobe—leggings might work with that upscale blazer, or that cardigan you've had forever might go well with those maternity trousers.

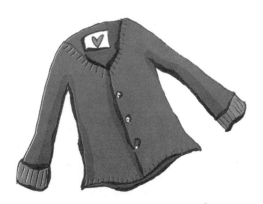

check those return policies

When you're purchasing maternity wear, look at those return policies before buying. Because you have such a limited amount of time in which to wear these clothes, you need to make sure they fit—and can go back if they don't! Most stores will let you return items for a full refund or store credit, but if you buy something on sale, you may be dismayed to find it unreturnable. When ordering online or through catalogs, be aware of the cost to ship something back to the store—many stores will let you return the item, but they won't pay for you to ship it back!

color your life

Don't just go black! You don't have to wear solely black when you're pregnant—no matter how slimming it is. You can also flaunt your love of color. You don't have to go crazy, but if you liked purple paisley shirts when you weren't pregnant, then go ahead and wear them now that you are.

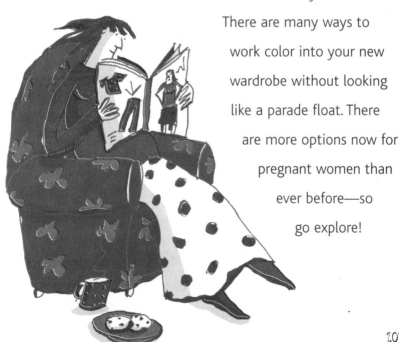

There are many ways to work color into your new wardrobe without looking like a parade float. There are more options now for pregnant women than ever before—so go explore!

tips on going out

Here are a few tips to help you prepare for an evening out.

🖐 Experiment with separates. Search your closet (or your best friend's) for any pieces you may have that you can combine to form an appropriate outfit. Favorite pairings are a black skirt with a cashmere sweater set, or slim black pants with a taffeta evening blouse or tunic. If you're going to wear all black, add a dash of color and luxury with a pashmina, cashmere, or silk wrap.

🖐 Play up your best features: work with styles that accentuate your arms and legs, because this will balance your beautifully expanding belly. Choose sleeveless tops or dresses—they create one long silhouette. When you're deciding between long and short hemlines, go for short and wear stockings that match your shoes so that your legs form slim, uninterrupted lines.

🖐 Visit a rental boutique if you have a black-tie event to go to and don't want to make do with what you have. It's the equivalent of a man renting a tuxedo for the night, so why not try it? You have nothing to lose!

Dress up your hair and makeup a notch. Emphasize your eyes with a shimmery shadow and two coats of mascara, and give your lips a swipe of gloss. Take a few extra minutes to blow-dry your hair with a round brush, then smooth a few drops of silicone-based serum over it for shine.

flatter your figure

Wear clingy pieces—anything that fits closely to your body looks cleaner, neater, and more flattering, says Liz Lange, owner of Liz Lange Maternity. Invest in a tapered skirt made from a high-quality stretchy material: cotton/Lycra for casual wear, or stretch wool or gabardine for a dressier look, says Lange. A knee-length style is best, because you look professional, but are still showing a little leg. And opt for slim-fitting pants with a boot-cut bottom—they're more figure flattering.

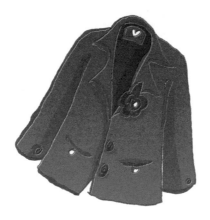

believe in the blazer

Wear your fitted jackets as long as you can, simply unbuttoning the bottom buttons for extra room, until you're finally forced to keep your jacket open. Then buy a maternity blazer, says Cherie Serota, cofounder of the Belly Basics clothing line. Look for one that's "unconstructed"—with no closures, so it just drapes over your belly, giving a fluid line. Dress it up with color and details. Wear shirts with a collar that will accentuate your collarbones and make your neck appear long—try a V-neck or boatneck.

stock up on stockings

During pregnancy, your legs are often your most valuable
asset, so don't be afraid to show them off! Choose stockings
that match your skirt or dress for a slim-line
monochromatic look: so, sheer black stockings
if you're wearing a black dress. If you're
suffering from varicose veins, you'll
probably want to choose opaque tights;
otherwise, show some skin. Queen-size
stockings can probably see you through
most of your term, but look for maternity
hosiery when they grow snug.

put your feet up

Most office chairs are not well designed for women and put pressure on a vein in the backs of your thighs. During pregnancy, this pressure translates into swollen legs and feet, even if you never leave your desk! While you're working, prop your feet up on a stool or box about 6–8 inches high (12–15 cm). And don't forget to get up and walk around after sitting at your desk for an hour so. On the other hand, if you have to stand at work, try to move around, or get a stool to rest one foot on.

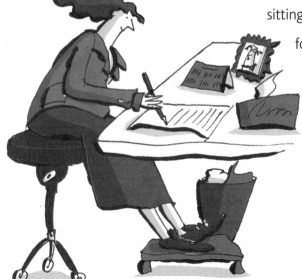

215

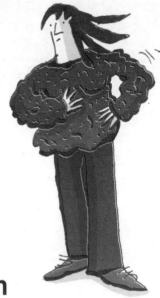

sensitive skin

Skin that never had any problem wearing wools and angoras may develop sensitivity to scratchy fabrics during pregnancy— particularly skin that's being stretched more than you ever thought it could be. Extra body heat contributes to this problem as well. Powders and lotions may help soothe itchiness, but you might have to give up your wools during the winter.

wicked accessories

Find an accessory that makes you feel wicked (don't fall into the trap of thinking wickedness is a luxury that only the single and childless among us can afford). One mom says, "Feeling wicked reminds us how we got to be parents in the first place! My 'wicked' accessory is toe rings, and the best I've found is through Toejam [*www.toejam.net*]—they even sell diamond-encrusted toe rings, and they are very comfy and sexy, and affordable."

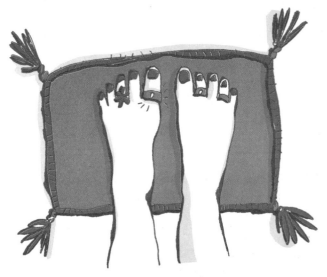

It Worked For Me ...

the medical stuff

Tests, tests, and more tests. If someone gives you a cup during these pregnant days, you're probably more likely to pee in it than pour yourself a drink! Don't worry. Although there are many tests and other medical issues to endure in pregnancy, there are good reasons for most of them.

You may find yourself, especially during your first pregnancy, not only worrying about every little thing, but inclined to take every test, read every medical manual, and consult your health-care provider constantly. The tips in this chapter often take the form of information on what you can expect on the medical side of pregnancy. All the moms I talked to said that what really freaked them out

the medical stuff

was when something unexpected happened—a test, a

medical term that wasn't properly explained, and so on—

and they gave me some examples. I've set

them down with as much

explanation as possible, in

the hope that some of

them will stem your

medical anxieties

at the source!

your primary care provider

Choosing your primary care provider is the most important medical decision you'll make during your pregnancy. It's also the toughest one to give advice on because women feel comfortable with different levels of medical intervention. You need to make sure your potential care provider agrees (at least on most points) with your philosophy of childbirth. These are the choices available:

Perinatologist: this is a doctor who specializes in high-risk pregnancy and works in a hospital setting, usually in conjunction with a Level III nursery.

Obstetrician: a doctor who specializes in pregnancy, birth, and gynecology, and who usually works in a hospital setting, though many are now starting up birth centers and a few do home births.

Family practitioner: another doctor who specializes in family care, including pregnancy and birth; usually works in combination with an obstetrician for surgical cases in a hospital or a birth center, as well as in home birth settings.

Nurse-midwife: a nurse with training in low-risk pregnancies and birth (about 90 percent of births fall into this category); works in conjunction with a doctor in home, hospital, or birth center settings.

Midwife: may have special training solely in midwifery and is trained to treat only low-risk pregnancies. She may or may not work with a doctor and usually practices in a home or birth center.

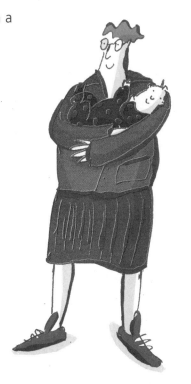

afp testing

AFP (alpha fetoprotein) testing is done to screen for neural-tube defects such as spina bifida and anencephaly. and has more recently attempted to predict the risks of Down syndrome.

It is a blood test taken from the mother in a lab, hospital, or the office of your practitioner, and is most sensitive when done at 15–17 weeks of gestation. Test results are usually given as ratios: for example, a risk of neural-tube defect of 1 in 500. There is no risk in the test itself, although, because of the risk of a false positive (when a baby is thought to have a problem, but is in fact healthy), AFP testing often leads to other, more invasive tests that do carry a risk to your pregnancy and your baby. As an alternative, ultrasound screening can also help determine your status with a bit less accuracy. I had AFP testing done with my first child and was given a falsely high result, which freaked me out completely. My child turned out just fine, and I opted

the medical stuff

out of the alternative amniocentesis (I was only 20 years old) and had an ultrasound instead. Do discuss this test thoroughly with your care provider to determine whether you really need it.

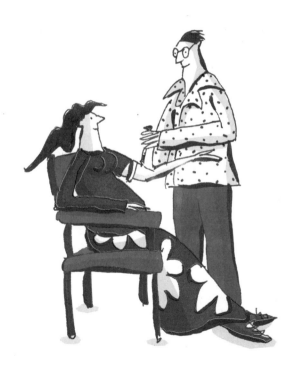

the medical stuff

amniocentesis

This test can be used to determine whether your baby has a
chromosomal disorder or fetal lung immaturity. A small needle is
pushed into the abdomen to the uterus to collect a sample of
amniotic fluid. Ultrasound is used to guide the needle away from
the baby and the placenta. Testing can be done from as early as
11 weeks, but more commonly done at 15–18 weeks, until the
end of pregnancy. Fetal lung immaturity is tested before the
decision is made to induce or let preterm labor continue (usually
after 34 weeks). If genetic disorders are detected, you will be
referred to a counselor for decision-making. If you are younger
than 35, most health-care providers will advise you to think
carefully about amniocentesis, since it carries a small risk of
miscarriage (between 1 in 200 and 1 in 400, according to the
Centers for Disease Control and Prevention).

chorionic villus sampling

CVS can be used to determine whether your baby has a chromosomal disorder. A small needle or catheter is placed either through the abdomen or through the vagina to collect a small sample of villi (membranous projections that form the beginnings of the placenta). Ultrasound is used to guide the instrument away from the baby and the placenta. CVS can be done as early as eight weeks, but is usually performed after ten weeks. There is a three to five percent miscarriage rate associated with this test, and some studies suggest there may be a slight increase in the number of limb deformities from amniotic banding syndrome (when amniotic fibrous brands wrap around vital part of the fetus). If genetic disorders are detected, you will be referred to a counselor for decision-making.

oral glucose tolerance testing

This test will determine whether you suffer from gestational diabetes or glucose intolerance of pregnancy. It can be done fasting or nonfasting, with blood drawn from a finger or from your veins. You may be asked to drink a special sugar-enhanced liquid, or to eat jelly beans or a specific breakfast, candy bar, etc. Your blood will then be tested for the level of glucose in it. This risk-free test (also known as OGTT) is usually offered to women around 28 weeks of gestation, although if you have a family history of diabetes or had gestational diabetes in a previous pregnancy, you may be tested earlier. Any reading above 140 will usually require further testing. If you "fail" the one-hour test, you will then be asked to take a three-hour glucose test; if you fail this, you will probably be sent to a nutritionist to learn ways to control your glucose levels through diet. You will also be given a plan for monitoring blood-sugar levels to assess your progress.

the medical stuff

I didn't fail the test, but I didn't pass—I was right on the line and so wasn't declared diabetic, but had to totally cut out candies (my soft spot) and other sugars from my diet for the last three months of my fourth pregnancy. My lovely husband made it up to me by bringing me Ben and Jerry's ice cream rather than flowers when I had our son!

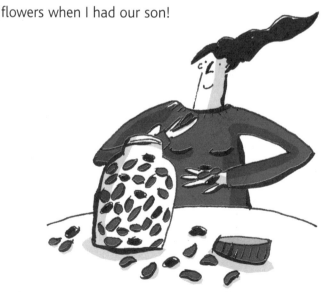

nonstress testing

This almost-risk-free test is generally used in cases where the mother is going past her assigned due date, to ensure fetal well-being; as a precaution after problems in a previous pregnancy; or because of high-risk factors. It is usually done in your practitioner's office, with fetal monitoring equipment hooked to your belly to record your baby's heart rate in conjunction with any uterine activity. You are asked to press a button when the baby moves, so that the heart rate can be seen in relationship to that movement. This test is typically done between weeks 38 and 42, although it can be used as early as the beginning of the third trimester. "Reactive" and "nonreactive" are usually the descriptions that result. Sometimes little ones don't cooperate by moving during the testing, so the mother is offered a drink of something sweet or carbonated to perk the baby up; if this doesn't work, a loud sound may be used to startle the baby into

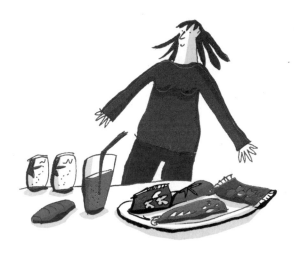

moving. Remember that babies can, and do, sleep *in utero*. If the baby is still not as responsive as your practitioner would like, you may be sent for a biophysical profile, a stress test, or even induction. I had this test in my first pregnancy when my son was two weeks overdue. It was uncomplicated, noninvasive, and put my mind at rest. I didn't want to be induced, so I just upped my walking time each day and went into labor within a couple of days.

stress testing

Stress testing establishes how well the baby will respond to the stress of contractions during labor. An injection of Pitocin is usually given and you are monitored via an electronic fetal monitor to see how your baby responds to contractions. This test is usually done at the very end of pregnancy, before an induction. The risks are that it may start labor or cause fetal distress. If the baby passes the test, you may be taken for other testing or left to wait for a natural labor to start. If your baby does not appear to deal well with contractions, you may be induced, or a cesarean birth may be decided upon.

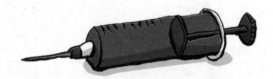

vaginal ultrasound

This is a comparatively unusual test that involves having a probe inserted into your vagina. I didn't have it during pregnancy, but much later when my last child was three years old, because of some pain and odd bleeding. It gives the doctor or midwife a view they can't get with a regular ultrasound, and is generally used only if you've had trouble in the past. Vaginal ultrasound can be done at any point in pregnancy, although in early pregnancy it is hard to detect anything. Although there is no proof that ultrasound is completely safe, leading bodies suggest that when the benefits outweigh the potential risks (usually left undefined), then this testing is appropriate. The best part? In a vaginal ultrasound (unlike ordinary ultrasound, *see pages 232–233*), you don't need to have a full bladder!

ultrasound testing

Ultrasound can give your practitioners a lot of valuable information. However, it is important to note that the routine use of ultrasound is questioned, even by the American College of Obstetricians and Gynecologists, in healthy, low-risk pregnancies. I had four low-risk pregnancies and took into account the pros and cons of the test. I opted for ultrasound because, well, I thought it would be cool to see the baby and because it gave me peace of mind to see the heart beating, the spine formed, the little fingers, and so on. The most frequent reasons for it are to date the pregnancy; to rule out ectopic (tubal) pregnancy; to check for fetal viability, particularly after bleeding or other complications; to screen for genetic defects or anomalies; to assist in genetic testing procedures such as amniocentesis and CVS. Testing can be done from around 18 weeks on, with an abdominal or vaginal probe (*see page 231*), depending on the

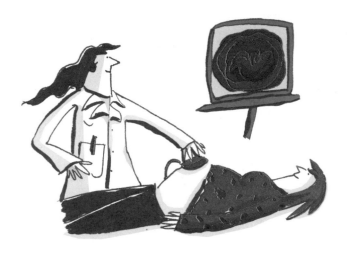

stage of the pregnancy and what your care providers are looking for. For abdominal ultrasound, a cold gel is applied to the abdomen to act as a conductor. The probe sends out high-frequency sound waves that bounce around the womb and are sent back as electrical signals, which are displayed as the image on the screen. You may be asked to have a full bladder for better viewing of the baby and uterus—a truly uncomfortable experience, although the view is worth it.

reducing the risk of diabetes

There are some commonsense measures you can take to reduce the risk of getting gestational diabetes. High-weight women should lose weight before pregnancy, but should not attempt to do so during pregnancy. Eat a diet low in simple sugars and high in fiber, and avoid processed foods (for example, eat whole-wheat toast and an orange rather than bran flakes and orange juice). Eat smaller meals more frequently, and eat a light breakfast. Moderate, regular exercise can lower blood sugar. To minimize the chance of getting a false positive on the OGTT (*see pages 226–227*), eat a high-carbohydrate diet for three days before the test; don't smoke during the test; and postpone it if you are ill, have an infection, or have been confined to bed, since all of these can elevate your blood sugar. (Eating jelly beans before the test is less likely to cause nausea than drinking concentrated glucose solution.) Visualization and relaxation

the medical stuff

techniques may help to reduce anxiety, which raises blood-sugar
levels. If diet does not control glucose values, try further dietary
adjustment or more exercise before agreeing to insulin therapy.
"I once heard it said that urine should be clear at least once a
day," Jill Stovsky, a registered dietician and diabetes educator
said. "Maybe this is an inaccurate saying, but very concentrated
urine that is dark in color means that you should be drinking
more. Every pregnant woman should drink about half a gallon
[2.25 l] of fluids every day, which should help to dilute and clear
up the urine."

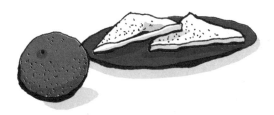

infectious diseases

During pregnancy, you need to minimize your exposure to infectious disease. Although a cold or flu won't harm your baby, some diseases can be dangerous. Measles can lead to fetal loss or premature birth; chickenpox and shingles can cause a variety of skin and other anomalies, as well as miscarriage, low birth weight, and stillbirth. Most women are immune, having had these diseases as children, but if you haven't, stay clear of those who are infectious and ask your health-care provider for advice.

Toxoplasmosis is the most talked-about disease. A fetus exposed to this may suffer from hydrocephalus, convulsions, and calcium deposits on the brain, although women exposed to the disease in the second half of pregnancy are less likely to have babies with such severe damage, and toxoplasmosis can be treated with antibiotics. If you have cats, you should avoid emptying the litter box while you're pregnant (or wear rubber gloves and a face mask

the medical stuff

or scarf if you have to do so), since the disease can be transmitted by contact with cat feces. It can also result from eating undercooked, raw, or cured meat during pregnancy. To avoid infections such as listeriosis, salmonella, and toxoplasmosis, you need to be scrupulous about hygiene when handling and heating food; refrigerate all cooked and chilled food and dairy produce; and avoid eating raw and undercooked meat and poultry, raw eggs, unwashed vegetables and salads, ripened soft cheeses, and pâté.

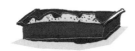

dental procedures

If you are having dental trouble, your dentist may need to take
an X-ray to get to the root (forgive the pun) of the problem.
The risk from dental X-rays is minimal, because you will be
shielded with a lead apron and the X-ray is taken well above
your abdomen, but make sure you tell your dentist you are
pregnant. Cavities, root canals, tooth extractions, and all the
other fun stuff can be done during pregnancy (ideally after
the first 12 weeks), provided a local anesthetic is used. If an
inhaled or intravenous anesthetic is recommended, consult your
healthcare provider and, if possible, put off the procedure until
after the baby is born. Dentists often prescribe antibiotics to
treat or prevent an infection. Dr. Marjorie Greenfield says,
"Barring any allergies, the penicillin and cephalosporin families of
medications are safe to take. Erythromycin, though sometimes
hard on the stomach, also is acceptable. Metronidazole (Flagyl),

which is sometimes used for serious abscesses, can be taken during pregnancy as well. Tetracycline should be avoided because it can affect the teeth and bones of a developing fetus."

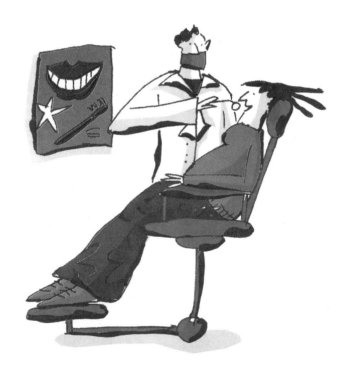

the rhesus factor

When your blood is tested to find out what blood type you have (A, B, AB, or O), you will also find out whether or not you have what is known as the "Rhesus (Rh) factor": some people (known as Rh-positive) have this antigen and others (Rh-negative) don't. As Dr. Marjorie Greenfield says, "Rh-negative is the only one of these blood groups that can cause a problem. It turns out that a Rh-negative mother can make antibodies (part of her immune system's response to invaders) against Rh-positive blood cells, even against those of her own baby. This is called Rh-sensitization. These antibodies have the potential to cross the placenta and attack the fetus's red blood cells, which in turn can cause low blood count (anemia), congestive heart failure, and even fetal death." Rhesus sensitization is preventable with medication known as Rh-immunoglobulin, which is given to all Rh-negative women whose fetuses might be Rh-positive.

The baby's blood type is then checked at birth, using blood obtained from the umbilical cord. If a woman does develop antibodies against Rh-positive cells (although this is now extremely rare), it will be detected in routine pregnancy blood-work. Rhesus sensitization (which can also occur in certain situations, such as after an abortion or miscarriage) usually doesn't hurt the baby in the first pregnancy, Greenfield says, because the mom can't make enough antibodies to cause severe problems. But the next pregnancy—and any that follow—can become very complicated if that fetus is Rh-positive. If possible, women who become Rhesus-sensitized should get their prenatal care from a high-risk obstetrical specialist (perinatologist), and should certainly seek guidance from their health-care provider.

hypertension

After the first few months of my first pregnancy, I became so used to having my blood pressure checked that I would wear clothes that would work well just for that purpose. I could never understand what was so important about my blood pressure, but it is a telltale sign that your practitioner needs to keep a close eye on. She is looking for what is known as pregnancy-induced hypertension, toxemia, or pre-eclampsia (*see pages 244–245*). Blood pressure generally decreases in the second trimester, and then goes back to its normal level during the third, but some women overshoot the mark and head higher than normal— triggering concern from their care provider. A blood pressure of 140/90 or above is typically considered to be elevated, Dr. Greenfield says. "Some women have blood pressures in that range even when not pregnant; for them, a 'high' blood pressure during pregnancy may be less of a concern, since they always run high. On the other hand, if a woman's blood pressure usually runs low, a rise in blood pressure during pregnancy (even if the pressure stays below 140/90) might still be considered elevated." A slightly elevated blood pressure is generally not a cause for alarm, but if this is accompanied by protein in the urine, swelling in the hands and face, or changes in certain blood tests, it could be indicative of pre-eclampsia.

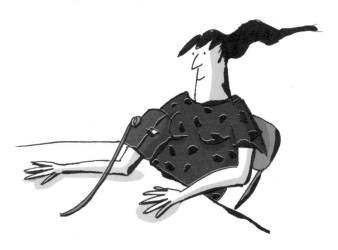

the medical stuff

pre-eclampsia

The symptoms of pre-eclampsia (also known as toxemia or pregnancy-induced hypertension) are different for every patient, and it is rare that a mom without previous blood-pressure issues would have a severe case of pre-eclampsia; however, the most serious cases develop into eclampsia, which may include seizures or temporary liver or kidney dysfunction. Some women who get pre-eclampsia have no indicating factors, other than that they are pregnant, but contributory factors include a woman over 40 or under 16, a history of high blood pressure, diabetes, or obesity. Many of the symptoms of pre-eclampsia can also occur in normal pregnancies and include swelling in your hands or feet; sudden weight gain (5 lb/2.25 kg in one week); a persistent headache; constant spots before your eyes; or pain in the upper abdomen. Women who experience any of these symptoms should tell their family practitioner right away to ensure they are not developing pre-eclampsia. Nothing has been shown to prevent pre-eclampsia in first-time, low-risk mothers. Some prevention strategies for higher-risk patients have been proposed, but none has found wide acceptance. The cure for pre-eclampsia is delivery, since it is a temporary condition that is resolved once the baby is born: in many cases, symptoms stop within minutes or hours. However, if it is too soon for your baby to be delivered, bed rest (*see pages 260–263*) and careful monitoring may be prescribed.

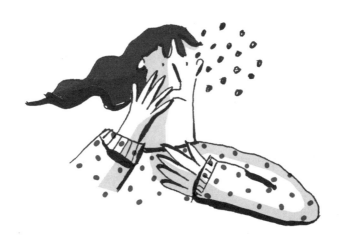

the medical stuff

sex during pregnancy

Many women, when they're not throwing up, find they have an increased interest in sex during pregnancy. For some, it's just the fact that the worry over birth control is eliminated; for others, it's caused by an increase in hormones. Some men find their pregnant wives very sexy, whereas others might be turned off, either by the weight gain or by the idea of hurting the baby, feeling "intrusive," or even thinking the baby "knows" what's going on. The best thing to do in these cases is to reassure your husband—or get your doctor or midwife to do so. Sex will not harm the baby, and, unless you have had trouble with placenta previa, bleeding, or a history of miscarriages, you can do it right up until your waters break. You won't hurt the baby by making love, even with your partner on top. The thick mucous plug that seals the cervix helps guard against infection; the amniotic sac and the strong muscles of the uterus also protect your baby.

Though your fetus may thrash around a bit after orgasm, it's because of your pounding heart, not because he knows what's happening or feels any pain. Normal oral sex won't harm you or your baby, and many consider it a good solution (particularly as you get larger) if intercourse is deemed uncomfortable or too risky for some reason.

However, blowing air into the vagina during pregnancy might cause an air embolism (obstructing a blood vessel) and could be dangerous for both you and your baby.

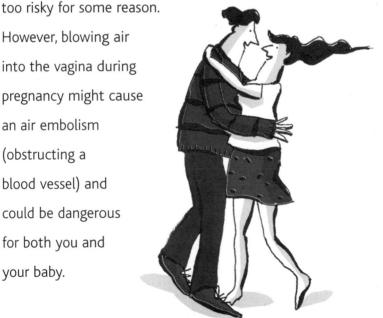

interesting positions

Now, what help would I be if I didn't give you a few safe ideas . . .
Here are some good positions—all recommended and proven
by other moms (and dads).

🖐 Lie sideways: having your partner on top demands
increasingly creative gymnastics as your tummy swells, but lying
partly sideways allows your partner to keep most of his weight
off your uterus.

🖐 Use the bed as a prop. Your bulge isn't an obstacle if you lie
on your back at either the side or the end of the bed, with your
knees bent and your bottom and feet perched at the very edge
of the mattress. Your partner can then either kneel or stand in
front of you.

🖐 Lie side by side in the spoons position, which allows for only
shallow penetration. Deep thrusts can become uncomfortable
as the months pass.

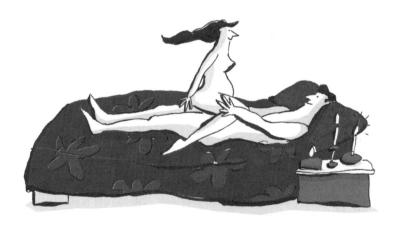 Get on top of your partner. This puts no weight on your abdomen and allows you to control the depth of penetration.

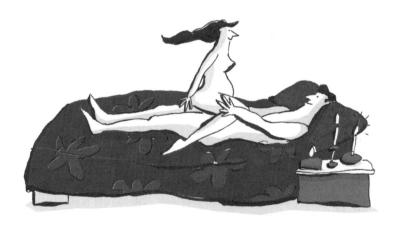 Enter from a sitting position, which also puts no weight on the uterus. Try sitting on your partner's lap as he sits on a (sturdy) chair.

working during pregnancy

Not very long ago, women who held jobs were expected to give them up as soon as the dipstick turned blue, but today you see pregnant women everywhere: holding down television anchor positions, teaching, running companies—you name it. Most women who continue working are experiencing a low-risk pregnancy, and there are situations where you might have to give up work or consider leaving earlier than expected. If you are exposed to toxic or chemical substances or infectious diseases at work, you should ask to be transferred to a less risky environment. If you have to stand for more than three or four hours at a time, you may want to stay at home or move to a different task. If you do a lot of lifting, stair- or ladder-climbing, or other strenuous activities, you might ask if there is some clerical work you can do for a while. If you work in a very hot, cold, or otherwise hostile environment, consider taking a seat at home. But you might be surprised by the number of employers who will let employees work from home, at least some of the time. If you present your boss with a plan (setting yourself up with a fax machine, extra phone line, high-speed Internet access, etc.), you may find him or her amenable to it—and it could help you once the baby is born. There are a number of books on working from home (I've listed several at the end of this guide), which can help you make the transition.

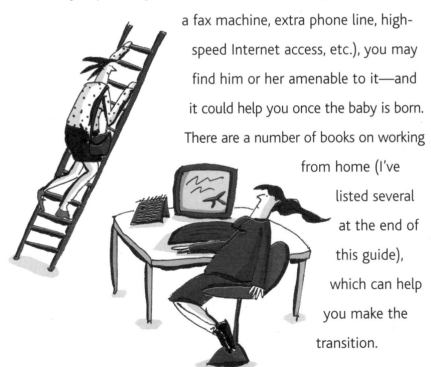

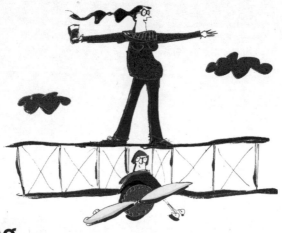

flying

As long as your pregnancy is normal, it's safe to go ahead and make travel plans as usual. Most expectant moms find that the second trimester (weeks 14–27) is a perfect time to travel. With morning sickness behind you, your energy levels high, and the chances of miscarriage low, you can enjoy the luxury of relaxing, sleeping in, and dining late with your partner. You can also take advantage of traveling light, with no car seat, stroller, diapers, or toys in tow. As long as you don't have medical complications, aren't carrying twins (or more), and haven't had any prior premature deliveries, you can fly on most airlines until the 36th week of pregnancy. Travel agents and airlines won't ask if you're pregnant when you book your seat, but you may be challenged at the check-in desk. From about 28 weeks of pregnancy, therefore, you will need a letter from your doctor confirming your due date and stating that you are unlikely to go into labor on the flight. Check your airline's policy on flying during pregnancy before you leave—and don't forget that it applies to your return trip, too.

comfort while flying

Here are some tips that should make flying more bearable:

🖐 Sitting anywhere for long periods of time can make your feet and ankles swell and your legs cramp. Keep your blood circulating by strolling up and down the aisle.

🖐 Do some simple stretches: sitting or standing, stretch your leg, heel first, then gently flex your foot to stretch your calf muscles. When sitting, rotate your ankles and wiggle your toes.

🖐 Flying during pregnancy can slightly increase your risk of thrombosis (blood clots) and varicose veins. Wearing support stockings (not panty hose, which increases your risk of developing thrush) when you fly will help keep your circulation flowing and relieve swollen veins. For maximum protection, put them on before you get out of bed in the morning and wear them all day.

🖐 If there's an empty seat next to you in the airplane, don't be afraid to put your feet up.

the medical stuff

🖐 Taking off your shoes may feel nice, but cabin pressure may make your feet swell during the flight, making your shoes tight when you put them back on. If your growing belly makes bending over a chore, slip-on shoes will make life easier, although they're usually less supportive for walking.

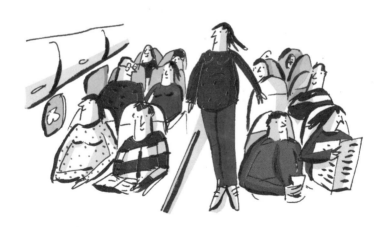

is flying harmful to baby?

There is no evidence that recreational flying is harmful to your growing baby. Cabin pressure won't affect your fetus; in fact, you're more likely to have problems flying in a small plane that doesn't have cabin pressure. Oxygen gets significantly thinner at high altitudes, which means that your body has to work hard to supply you—and your baby—with sufficient amounts. Air stewardesses make hundreds of flights each year, and although female flight attendants may be grounded during the first trimester of pregnancy as a precautionary measure, doctors agree that the risk to women who fly only occasionally is tiny.

could I be carrying twins?

Perhaps, although the most common reason for measuring larger
than you should is that your conception date isn't what you
thought it was. Signs of twins are a sizeable weight gain early on
or more than one heartbeat being heard. Most people find out
they're carrying twins at their first ultrasound scan. The usual
pregnancy symptoms are likely to be more severe—particularly
morning sickness. Other common problems include an inability to
sleep, fatigue, general discomfort and pain, swollen hands and feet,
and difficulty in moving about. Women go into premature labor
(before 37 weeks) in nearly half of twin pregnancies. Reaching
38 weeks increases the odds of babies being born healthy.

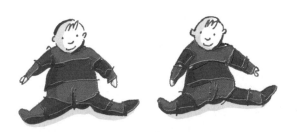

pee again?

At antenatal appointments, your midwife will use a dipstick to check for protein and sugar in your urine sample. The presence of protein in your urine (proteinuria) gives information about how your kidneys are working. Low amounts of protein are not uncommon, and may simply mean that your kidneys are working harder than they did before pregnancy. Your body may be fighting a minor infection, and the midwife may send your urine sample for analysis, to establish whether you have an infection, and of what type; you may then be prescribed antibiotics.

At the next appointment, the midwife will establish if there is still protein present, and whether the amount has increased. Increased proteinuria may be an indication that you are developing pre-eclampsia (*see pages 244–245*), one of the serious conditions of pregnancy, affecting the health of both mother and baby. A combination of raised blood pressure, worsening proteinuria, and swelling of the fingers, feet, and face suggests pre-eclampsia, although sometimes only one of these symptoms is present. If your urine sample has higher levels of protein, you will be referred for further tests: usually a 24-hour urine collection to measure exactly how much protein you are excreting, plus a blood sample to check on your liver function. You will probably be asked to stay in the hospital for these tests, although you may be able to negotiate on this.

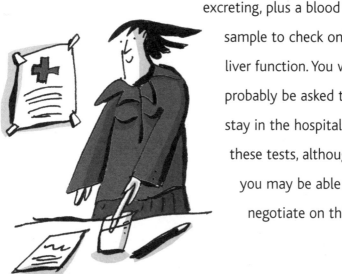

the medical stuff

surviving bed rest

The term "bed rest" can be a sentence or a savior. Either way, it will be tougher than you think. The first thing to do is find out from your care provider exactly how much bed rest you need—is it to be complete, with only trips to the bathroom allowed? Or can you do some things around the house and stay downstairs for a certain number of hours? Here are some tips from other moms to help you get through.

✋ Stick to a schedule: even if you have to stay in bed all day, you'll feel better if you feel you've accomplished something. So, after you wake up, change into comfortable clothes and plan what to do for the day.

✋ Catch up on correspondence or read your favorite author's latest novel while you can—let's face it, you'll be too busy after the baby arrives.

✋ Try these time-passers: organize photo albums; devour books, magazines, and newspapers; contact your job about your maternity-leave benefits; fill out health insurance paperwork for your baby in advance; designate a guardian for your child and have your lawyer draft a new will; and watch rented videos or taped TV shows.

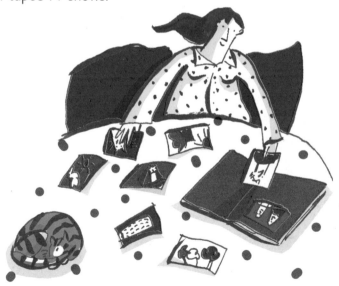

more tips on bed rest

Here are other ideas from pregnant moms who've been on bed rest.

🖐 Stock up: just because you're on your back doesn't mean you have to be unprepared. You can fully stock your baby's nursery and layette by phone or the Internet. Order all the items you think you'll need for the first three months—including diapers! Online pharmacies often carry a wide variety of baby-care items, which they'll deliver right to your door.

🖐 Don't be afraid to ask visitors, friends, and family for help with household chores, errands, or meal preparation. Create a task list so that when someone does offer help, you can assign him or her a task. Visits from your friends and family can boost your spirits—just make sure they come at a time that's convenient for you.

🖐 Become a parenting expert—there are plenty of web sites to answer your parenting and children's health questions. If you feel

the medical stuff

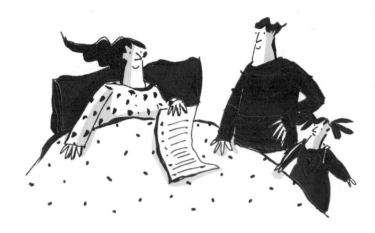

uncomfortable reading about high-risk pregnancy issues,
learn about breast-feeding or how to encourage your child's
development. And the Internet is a great place to find support
from other moms on bed rest—message boards and chat rooms
are good sources of tips and advice.

☝ Support your support person. You're probably relying heavily
on your partner now to do household chores, child care, and
errands. Make sure you show your appreciation—you can always
order a nice gift by phone or online!

about premature labor

Deborah M. Bash, director of the Nurse-Midwifery Education Program at Georgetown University in Washington, DC, says that the usual length of a pregnancy is 38–40 weeks after the first day of the last menstrual period. Premature or preterm labor is defined as labor occurring between 20 and 37 weeks. Estimates suggest that 6–10 percent of all births in the United States occur between the 20th and 37th week of pregnancy. Smoking (which has a well-established association with poor outcomes of pregnancy, including the risk of miscarriage), poor nutritional habits, drug and alcohol abuse, and other poor health practices during pregnancy increase the risk of early delivery and the birth of stillborn or sick infants. Unfortunately, it is difficult to predict which women are at risk. Sometimes women mistake a certain type of contraction for labor. As early as six weeks into all pregnancies, the uterus, which is a large muscle, begins to

contract rhythmically. These contractions (known as Braxton
Hicks contractions, *see pages 318–319*) are usually irregular and
painless, and because they do not normally cause the cervix
to dilate, they do not threaten the pregnancy. Braxton Hicks
contractions that increase in frequency and intensity toward
the end of pregnancy are sometimes referred to as "false labor"
contractions. Women are not usually aware of cervical dilation
(the stretching and opening of the entrance to the uterus),
which can be measured only by a health practitioner during
a pelvic examination.

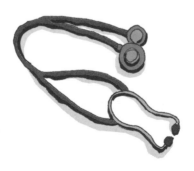

what to do

If you think you are experiencing premature labor and are getting contractions (either painful or painless ones) that occur more than four times an hour, or that are less than 15 minutes apart, Deborah Bash recommends reporting this activity to your doctor or midwife. Be prepared to answer the following questions: When did the discomfort start? What is the type and frequency of the contractions? What were you doing when the symptoms began? Do you have any other signs or symptoms, such as

- menstrual-like cramps that come and go
- abdominal cramps with or without diarrhea
- backache that is dull and may radiate around or toward the abdomen
- an increase in vaginal discharge or a noticeable change in color
- pelvic pressure that is constant or intermittent?

While you are waiting to hear back from your care provider, sit down with your feet elevated and drink a glass of water or juice. Try to relax, take deep breaths, and distract yourself with television or the radio. Many times, Braxton Hicks feel real, until you actually go into labor—then the difference becomes quite obvious. If these contractions are very different from the usually abdominal tightening of Braxton Hicks, then you may very well be in labor.

It Worked For Me . . .

the second trimester

By the time you reach the second trimester, at around 14 weeks, the morning sickness and extreme fatigue will hopefully be coming to an end. If they're not, they soon will—I can almost promise! But as your energy is increasing, so is your belly, and this can bring on other weirdnesses that you're not quite ready for: stretch marks, itchiness, and all kinds of fun stuff.

Here are tips about some of the biggest (and smallest) issues facing you in the second trimester—and some of the excitements as well, like those first flutters in your belly (often described as "butterflies"). It's a wonderful time when you really start to feel pregnant,

instead of as if you've just got the flu, and you don't yet
have the aches and pains of the third
trimester. And your fetus is now
beginning to look like a real baby,
with eyebrows and eyelashes,
and even ears to tune in to your
conversations. Don't feel silly
if you start to talk to your
stomach—just think how
well your baby will know
your voice when he or
she finally appears.

stretch marks

Let's begin with the stuff that's really going to bug you: good old stretch marks. Now, I know many women who never got one stretch mark (and I try not to hate them), but there are some of us who are going to get them no matter how many lotions we use. I had four babies and my stretch marks got worse with each one: on the front of my belly, my sides, even a couple on my thighs, although they have softened over the years. First of all, here are some facts:

🖐 *Striae gravidarum*, or stretch marks, appear in 50–90 percent of all pregnant women, usually showing up in the later half of pregnancy. Although the majority will be on the lower abdomen, they may also occur on the thighs, hips, buttocks, breasts, and arms.

🖐 They commonly manifest as small depressions in the skin, and tend to be pinkish in light-skinned women, and lighter than the surrounding skin in dark-skinned women.

🖐 Although stretch marks themselves are not painful, the stretching of the skin may cause a tingling or itchy sensation.

🖐 Many people swear by certain creams; others say there's not much you can do about stretch marks—you'll either get them or not, although there are factors that predispose you to them. If your mom or sister has them, guess what? Rapid or excessive weight gain will make them worse; well-hydrated and healthy skin stretches better than poor skin; and African-American women get them less often.

🖐 So, what can you do about them? Well, stretch marks do fade after the birth, becoming silver lines, like mine. Most women don't think about them much, but others want them removed, and new techniques (including laser options) are being developed all the time. Talk to your dermatologist or plastic surgeon if you are concerned.

other skin issues

🖐 A skin condition known as the "mask of pregnancy," or chloasma, occurs when melanotropin is secreted in greater quantities than usual, causing pigmentation to occur over the nose, cheeks, and forehead of an expectant mom. Although it is not caused by sunlight, this will aggravate the symptoms. About 45–70 percent of women will get chloasma, beginning in the fourth or fifth month of pregnancy, but it will fade after the birth. Most women use makeup to cover the blemishes if they become very noticeable.

🖐 The *linea nigra* is a darker line extending from the pubic bone to the top of the uterus, which usually shows up for first-time moms around the third month, although multiparous women (those who have given birth to more than one child) will often see it manifest earlier. Don't believe the rumors that it means a baby boy is on the way.

Spider veins commonly appear on the face, neck, chest, arms, and legs, and are caused by increased estrogen levels in your body. They are often star shaped and slightly raised, pale blue, and do not turn white with pressure; 65 percent of Caucasian women and 10 percent of African-American women get spider veins, which again usually fade after the birth. For me, this was just another entry in the category of "get over it."

Palmar erythema is a similar mottled or reddening of the palms, again caused by raised estrogen levels. About 60 percent of Caucasian women and 35 percent of African-Americans suffer.

Discuss any skin issue new to you with your care provider.

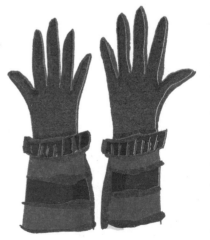

acne

Thought pimples were a teenage thing? Think again. Although many women find that the hormones of pregnancy actually relieve their acne and leave them with that "glowing" skin, others discover that their skin is more oily than usual and susceptible to acne breakouts. (Yes, that would be me—again!) Go back in your mind to those good old high-school days and try to make sure you drink plenty of water, wash your face, and avoid foods that cause you to break out. I found that wiping my face down with a little rubbing alcohol on an absorbent cotton

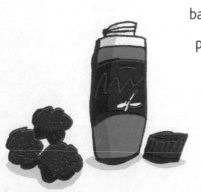

ball helped to dry my pimples out. There are also some great face washes containing microbeads or walnut shells, which may help.

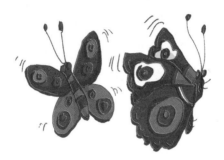

feeling baby move

Although you can expect to feel your baby's movements at some point in the second trimester, you shouldn't necessarily assume that Junior will be doing somersaults by week 16, according to Ann Douglas, a Canadian writer on pregnancy and a mother of four. More often than not, the first flutters aren't felt until weeks 18–22, although slimmer moms and experienced mothers may detect them a bit earlier. The location of the placenta can also affect how much movement you feel (if it's at the front of your uterus, it will tend to cushion Junior's gymnastic performances!).

a couple of myths

Ever heard that you can tell the sex of your baby by mixing Drano with your urine? According to childbirth educator and doula Robin Weiss, "The Drano test supposedly can detect something in a pregnant woman's urine that will change the color of the Drano to indicate the gender of the baby. However, this is absolutely false. In addition, I must warn you that it is extremely dangerous to mix urine and Drano. When they did studies at medical school on this test, they wore chemical masks and did them under chemical hoods because of the possibility of fumes and explosion. Currently we know of nothing that is excreted in a pregnant woman's urine to enable us to predict the gender of her baby."

Another myth is being able to predict the sex of your child by the heart rate. The common belief was that 140+ meant a girl and below 140 a boy. The truth? The heart rate of your baby fluctuates as he or she grows and moves. Heart rates start out slower, and then by 8–10 weeks run in the range of 170–200 BPM (beats per minute). As you approach midpregnancy, the average heart rate is 120–160 BPM. If your baby moves, his or her heart rate goes up, just as your own does with movement. However, none of these rates is related to the sex of your baby. A recent study actually showed there is no correlation between gender and fetal heart rate.

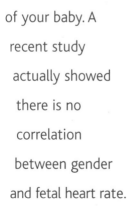
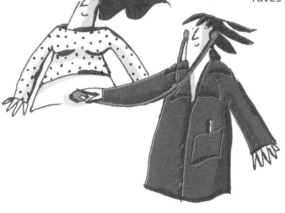

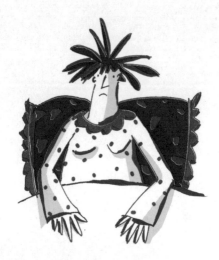

disturbing dreams

Waking up in the middle of the night from a horrifying dream about your baby may be terrifying, but it is quite normal. Sleep researchers pin much of the blame on pregnancy hormones, which can affect your sleep patterns. Fortunately, such dreams don't indicate a problem with your baby's health. You're no more at risk of giving birth to a baby with health problems than someone who dreams of picture-perfect Gerber babies.

a ripping sensation?

The sensation you may be experiencing is round ligament pain, caused by the sudden stretching of the round ligaments (the two large ligaments that attach your uterus to your pelvis). It tends to be at its worst between the 14th and 20th weeks of pregnancy, when your uterus is heavy but not yet large enough to rest any of its weight on the pelvic bones—which typically happens during the latter half of the second trimester. Although round ligament pain can be alarming (and at times even painful), it's not something serious to worry about.

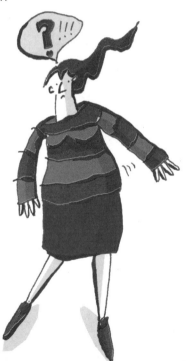

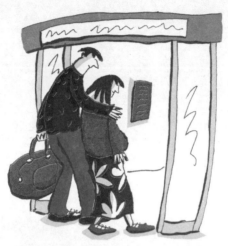

a tight abdomen

You're out for a walk and your abdomen goes hard and rigid—it doesn't really hurt, but it feels very strange. This sensation can be uncomfortable, but generally isn't a cause for concern. That said, it's good to familiarize yourself with the signs of premature labor (*see page 266*) so you can recognize preterm labor contractions. If in doubt, err on the side of caution. Better to show up at the labor ward with a "false alarm" than to give birth unprepared.

loss of symptoms

The early part of the second trimester is a bit of a no-woman's-land when it comes to pregnancy symptoms. The first-trimester fatigue and nausea have probably begun to subside, and you're unlikely to be experiencing a lot of fetal movement at this stage. Get in touch with your family practitioner or midwife to talk about any concerns. Something as simple as hearing your baby's heart beat can help to reassure you that everything's proceeding according to plan.

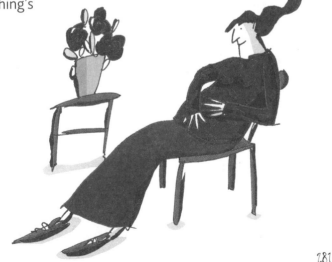

I'm losing my mind!

One minute you're happy, the next you're crying at television commercials. Plus, you're now forgetting everything: why you walked into the room, your keys, a meeting. Don't worry; I often said that I expelled part of my brain with the birth of each child! This is normal . . . but freaking out about it will only make it worse. Try to laugh it off—even when you feel like you want to cry.

Reducing some of the stress in your life can help, and making lists is useful. If you're worried you'll do things like leave the stove on, get into the routine of checking it before you head to bed. It will save you waking up in the middle of the night saying, "Oh my God, did I . . . ?"

that itchy feeling

About 20 percent of all pregnant women have some kind of generalized skin itchiness. Hormones and your stretching skin—especially over your belly—are probably to blame, but consult your doctor if there is excessive itching, the skin looks jaundiced, or to rule out scabies, atopic eczema, or urticaria. Apply moisturizer or try a warm oatmeal bath to soothe tingling skin. Heat rash can intensify the itching, so wear loose cotton clothing and avoid going out in the heat of the day.

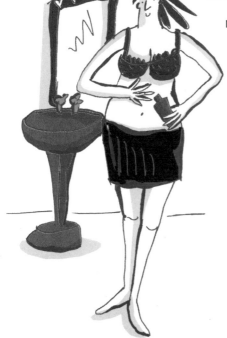

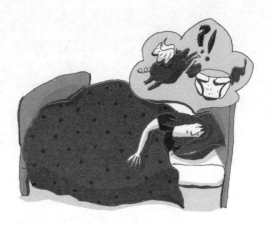

second-trimester sleep

Enjoy it while you can! By now, your body will be adjusting to its hormonal changes, since the influx of progesterone has tapered to a steady drizzle. So you should be feeling less tired than you did in the first months and able to sleep more peacefully. Bear in mind, though, that the quality and quantity of your sleep still won't be as good as they were before you were pregnant, and you may be affected by snoring (*see pages 288–289*), congestion (*see page 60*), leg cramps (*see page 110*), or vivid dreams (*see page 278*).

make the most of your energy

At the same time, your sense of renewed energy may mean
that you don't want (or need) the extra shut-eye. Life's so unfair!
While you're feeling more energetic and getting a reasonable
night's sleep, start exercising regularly (see the chapter on
exercise for a wealth of ideas, some of which should appeal to
you). Exercise will boost your mental and physical health, and
in turn help you sleep more soundly at night.

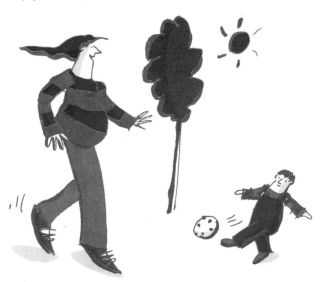

nosebleeds

Inconvenient and even embarrassing as they may be, nosebleeds are a perfectly normal symptom of pregnancy. Your increased blood supply puts pressure on your nose's delicate veins, and the membranes inside your nose may also swell and dry out, especially in winter. These changes can cause those veins to rupture quite easily, bringing about minor nosebleeds. When your nose bleeds, remain seated and put pressure on the bleeding nostril for at least four minutes. (Don't lie down, or the blood may run into your stomach, which might cause nausea or vomiting.) Consult your doctor if you frequently have heavy nosebleeds, or if the above measures don't stop the bleeding. To avoid nosebleeds try the following: avoid nasal dryness, especially in winter time or in dry climates, by coating the edges of your nose with Vaseline (or you could use a humidifier inside your house); blow your nose gently, since aggressive blowing can lead to nosebleeds; drink extra fluids to help keep all your tissues (including the mucous membranes) well hydrated. Although nosebleeds are annoying, they are a temporary problem that is likely to disappear after you have your baby.

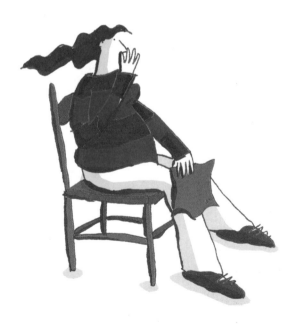

becoming a snorer?

As you enter your second trimester, you may find yourself snoring for the first time in your life. You—and your partner— may be less than thrilled by this new development, but take heart, because there's a good chance that you'll stop snoring after your baby is born. The cause of your midnight melodies is swollen nasal passages. During pregnancy, an increase in progesterone may cause the soft tissues of the nasal passages to swell and partially block the airways. Alternatively, your airways may be naturally narrow or, if you have extra tissue in the back of your throat, pregnancy-induced swelling or fluid retention may block your airways. According to a sleep survey, about 30 percent of moms-to-be start to snore during this time. If you have a severe nasal blockage, then you risk developing sleep apnea, which is characterized by loud snoring and periods of arrested breathing. You can help control your snoring by sleeping on your side rather than on your back; or by wearing a nasal strip (available at most pharmacies) to keep your nostrils wide open. Avoid alcohol, tobacco, and sleeping pills, because all three can make the airways more likely to close.

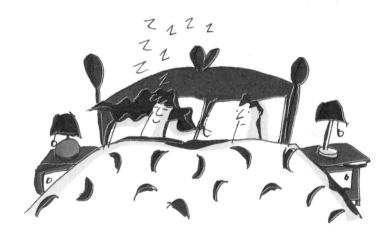

a pain in the butt—literally

Sciatica is pain originating from the sciatic nerve, which runs from the lower back, through the buttocks, and down the back of each leg. It can manifest as a shooting, burning pain in the lower back, thigh, leg, or foot, as pins and needles, or numbness. It may come and go, affect just one side, or be so severe that every movement is excruciating. I had terrible sciatica during my pregnancies (but I have had it all my life), and it is not unusual to get it in your second or third trimester, although it often goes away after the baby is born. For bad pain, I received deep heat massage, but I eventually invested in an electric massager with a heat setting. Exercises to help strengthen your pelvic floor and abdominal muscles are also quite useful. So is acetaminophen, but consult your care provider before using it. Some women have great success with a chiropractor, but make sure he or she is experienced in treating pregnant women. Other helpful ideas:

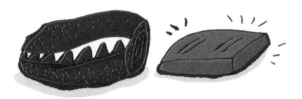

✋ Keep your back as straight as possible at all times: try not to stick out your belly or arch your back.

✋ Apply a heat or ice pack to the painful area for 10 minutes.

✋ Wear soft, flat shoes to help prevent jarring of the spine as you walk.

✋ Avoid sitting still for long periods.

✋ Listen to your body and stop doing whatever is causing pain.

✋ During the latter stages of pregnancy, a TENS machine is safe to use to help control pain (*see page 398*).

✋ When seated, use a small cushion or a rolled-up towel behind your back; use pillows and cushions to support your belly in bed.

✋ Avoid heavy lifting—if you do have to lift anything, bend from your knees and keep your back straight.

tossing and turning

Getting—and staying—comfortable in bed may be one of your greatest challenges during pregnancy, particularly if you're used to sleeping on your stomach or back, since both positions present problems. During your first trimester, tender breasts may prevent you from sleeping on your stomach, and as your belly grows, lying facedown will become increasingly uncomfortable. Sleeping on your back puts the full weight of your uterus on your back, intestines, and the inferior vena cava (the vein that transports blood from your lower body to your heart); it can also increase your risk of developing backaches and hemorrhoids, poor digestion, impaired breathing and circulation, and even low blood pressure. In your first trimester, get into the habit of sleeping on your left side. This benefits your baby by maximizing the flow of blood and nutrients to the placenta; it also helps your kidneys to expel waste products from your body more efficiently, which in turn reduces swelling in your ankles, feet, and hands. Try curling up or stretching out on your left side with extra pillows between your legs, under your belly, and behind your back for support (and return to that position if you wake up and find yourself on your stomach or back)—you can buy special maternity pillows, though your usual pillows may work just as well. Later on, you may find that wearing a sleeping bra and a maternity belt will make you more comfortable. Finally, if lying on your side puts too much pressure on your hips, buy a piece of soft foam to put on top of your mattress and under the sheet, for added comfort and air circulation.

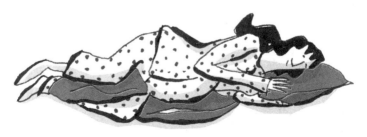

caring for your teeth

There is an old wives' tale that says a woman loses a tooth for each child she carries. This isn't exactly true, but being pregnant can increase dental issues. Gingivitis is inflammation of the gums and is a fairly common problem. It can result from increased blood flow to the gums caused by pregnancy hormones. If you are also bruising easily, have frequent or heavy nosebleeds, or are bleeding from anywhere else, let your health-care provider know. Brush your teeth with a soft-bristle toothbrush at least twice a day to help prevent cavities, and floss regularly. Adults should have their teeth cleaned every six months, but pregnant women might consider having it done more frequently (like every three).

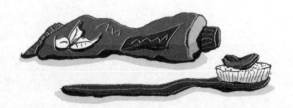

bank on it, baby

One mom says that perhaps the most important item to get for your baby's room is a piggy bank, as soon as you find out you're expecting. Drop your spare change in whenever you can, and this becomes a foolproof way to start baby's first savings—even if you think you can't afford to save right now. When you have compiled a decent amount, look into ways to invest it for baby's future. After all, your baby will be an adult one day, and he or she will be thrilled to find that your frugality has paid off and there's some cash to help him or her with college.

can I buy the stuff yet?

Buying all the new gear is one of the best parts of being pregnant—until you watch your checkbook balance drop like a rock in a pond at each new expenditure. No one ever told me that babies were this expensive before they even showed up! Here are some tips from other frugal moms on how to get the stuff you need and still keep a little cash in the bank: maybe for that last date with your partner before you become permanent homebodies! Yard sales, thrift stores, and consignment stores are good places to find infant and toddler toys, gear, and furniture. Here prices can be as low as one quarter of the normal price for such things as rattles, mobiles, and squeaky toys. Used strollers and other travel accessories will typically save you at least half of the retail price. But you do need to be careful: always ask for a demonstration to make sure electronic goods actually work. And check to see that items haven't been recalled—this is especially important with car seats, which must meet strict safety guidelines today. You can find this information online at the U.S. Consumer Product Safety Commission (*www.cpsc.gov*) and in the BabyCenter.com recall database (*www.babycenter.com/recall*).

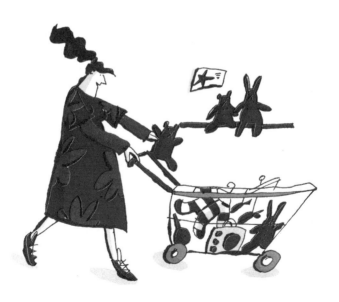

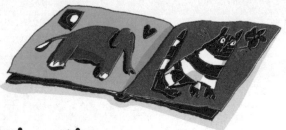

shopping tips

🖐 Ask thrift-store managers when their trucks come in, one mom suggests. Many get deliveries on certain days, so go that evening or the next morning for the best selection (Monday mornings are good because people donate over the weekend).

🖐 Don't forget used bookstores, another mom adds. You can get great deals on children's classics and board books; used music stores can be stocked with cheap treasures, too.

🖐 Many stores sell the bulk of their inventory (especially toys) during the Christmas season and then everything goes on sale, usually at drastically reduced prices, so buying birthday presents and next year's gifts after January 1 can save you lots of money.

stick with the basics

When you go to baby stores, you'll see all kinds of strollers, walkers, bouncers, car seats, and carriers. Remind yourself to buy only what you need (*see pages 304–307*). Your baby probably doesn't need the latest $300 designer stroller, and buying low-end basics can save you hundreds of dollars. You won't spot any Chippendale dressers at stores that specialize in flat-pack furniture, but you will find sturdy basics at affordable prices. The catch? You often have to assemble the furniture yourself, but anyone who can use a screwdriver and wood glue can usually manage.

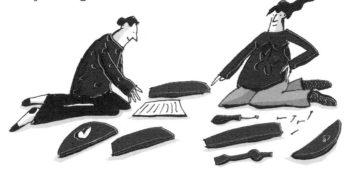

outlet centers and floor samples

A trip to the furniture outlet center of a large department store can save you serious money. This furniture often has small nicks or imperfections, so it can't be sold for full price. But, with a coat of white paint or some cute teddy bear stencils, you can turn a dresser into the perfect centerpiece for the nursery. And don't overlook floor samples, one mom says. They're often cheaper than new products because they've suffered a little wear and tear, but the best part is that they're already put together.

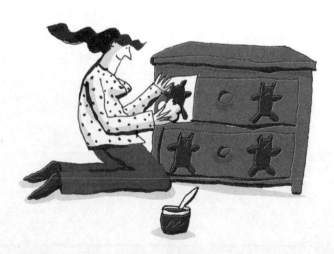

stash those diapers

"One of the best pieces of advice I got from a friend," one mom says, "was to start buying diapers as soon as you find out you're pregnant." Having a nice, large stash of these lessens the shock to the bank balance once baby arrives. Buy just one pack or so of the newborn size (since you may have a bigger baby), and mostly packs of sizes 1 and 2. And don't ever buy brand-name diapers without a coupon—

you can easily shave $1–3 off the price with newspaper coupons, and by shopping when the discount stores have their monthly sale on the megapack size.

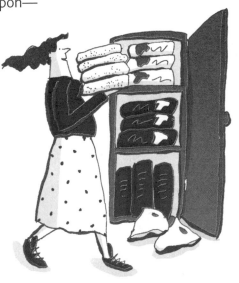

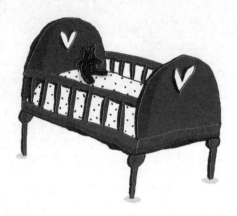

raid attics and basements

For those of you lucky enough to be from a family of pack rats, pick through your parents'/in-laws'/friends' attics or basements for old baby furniture, strollers, car seats, and so forth. You can also check shoppers' guides, consignment shops, and flea markets. A word of warning, though. Take a good look at crib slats; the rails should be no more than 2⅜ inches (5.5 cm) apart, or your baby's head could get trapped. And car seats are constantly being improved, so it's safest not to use one that's more than about two years old.

wait a bit

"Don't buy in all yellow or white," one mom says. If you don't know your baby's sex, resist the urge to buy neutral colors. If you choose to find out your baby's sex ahead of time, you won't know until at least the 20th week, so hold off until then, and you can buy in pink or blue (if you wish). And wait until after your shower (which may not be until the third trimester) to buy baby items, since babies bring out people's generosity. Let your family and friends know you are hoping to get diapers, formula, and other essential items, because this will free up money in your budget. This way at least you don't get 50 baby grooming kits.

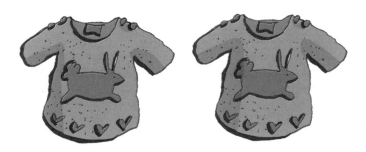

necessities vs. luxuries

You probably don't need a lot of the items you think you need, so here's a breakdown that may help.

🖐 Necessity: a crib. This is a big-ticket item with a big price tag. If you're tempted to get a used model or a hand-me-down, make sure the crib adheres to current safety standards.

🖐 Luxuries: a cradle or bassinet (compact and portable, but babies outgrow them very quickly and can sleep in a crib from day one); a co-sleeper (an infant bed that fits securely against your bed—the safest choice if you're planning to have a family bed).

🖐 Necessity: well-fitting crib sheets and mattress. It's important to use sheets specifically designed for cribs, which fit tightly around a firm, snugly fitting mattress.

🖐 Luxuries: matching bedding sets (bumper pads are cute, but not necessary for baby's comfort; quilts and pillows can't be used in the crib for safety reasons); a mobile (a wind-up musical version can be a great soothe-to-sleep tool, but must conform to safety standards).

Necessity: a changing pad with sloped sides and a safety strap, which you can set on top of a regular waist-high chest of drawers so that it is at the right height.

Luxuries: a changing table (although it may be worth the investment if you're planning to have more than one child, or if it converts to another use); extra covers for the changing pad.

Necessity: a comfy chair for feeding times. You should have a special seat (a rocking chair, recliner, or armchair) where you can put up your feet and relax during those countless feedings.

Luxuries: a glider chair (expensive, and very nursery specific, but some moms love them); a special nursing pillow and footstool (you can improvise with regular pillows and footstools).

more necessities and luxuries

🖐 Necessity: a diaper pail. If you want a budget option, consider a simple diaper pail and a supply of plastic grocery bags.

🖐 Luxuries: a fancy diaper pail (many parents swear by their Diaper Genies); a diaper stacker; a baby-wipe warmer (a nice touch, though they sometimes cause the wipes to dry out).

🖐 Necessity: a baby tub or tub/sink liner. Baby bathtubs are not too expensive, but if you're looking to save money, consider a tub or sink liner—a thick sponge that cushions the baby. And a bath thermometer is inexpensive and has a big safety payoff.

🖐 Luxuries: hooded towels (handy, cozy, but not essential); baby washcloths (any soft cloth can be used).

🖐 Necessity: a car seat (*see page 297*).

🖐 Luxuries: car-seat toys; a sunshade (often provides only a tiny patch of protection for baby, so look for a big one); extra mirrors for parents to look at baby (these can be distracting for drivers).

✋ Necessity: a stroller or travel system. Consider a combo car-seat-stroller travel system (especially for suburban lifestyles with lots of driving), or save up for a well-made umbrella stroller.

✋ Luxuries: a fully reclinable carriage stroller, all-terrain or jogging stroller.

✋ Necessity: a front carrier, sling, or infant carrier. Front carriers and slings free up your hands, are great for baby-parent bonding, and are very packable, and an infant carrier often doubles as a car seat and/or part of a travel system.

✋ Luxuries: a backpack-style carrier (you can't carry a newborn baby this way); a special fleece cover (nifty, but you could always use a blanket instead).

life insurance

Debra Jo Immergut, a financial writer at *Parents* magazine, suggests considering term insurance. For most people, term insurance provides the most life coverage for the least cost. Because of the many variables (including your age and that of your children), there is no hard-and-fast rule concerning how much coverage to buy, but experts often suggest an amount equal to five times your annual salary. Check to see what life insurance your employer offers. Many companies provide term policies equal to one year's salary; coverage can often be increased by paying an extra premium. And consider insuring a stay-at-home parent. He or she should have enough life insurance to cover child-care costs, since, in the event of his or her death, the working spouse would probably need to hire a caregiver.

wills

Immergut says that every parent needs a will, because it allows you to name guardians for your kids. Otherwise, if something happened to you and your spouse, your child could end up as a pawn in a custody fight, or be raised by relatives whose parenting style might be at odds with your own. Why take the chance? Specify how you'd like your assets distributed. Even if you're just scraping by, your home, insurance proceeds, retirement contributions, and employee benefits could add up to a substantial estate. If you die without a valid will, state law will determine who gets everything—which can create big problems for survivors, and high fees to state-appointed administrators.

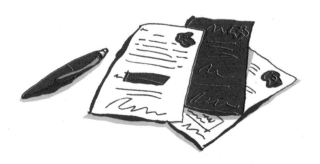

tips for dads

Dads are expectant, too, but often feel left out because so much attention is focused on the mom-to-be. Here are some suggestions that dads have said help them to feel involved:

☙ Rub her feet. Doing a hand or foot massage can help relieve tension and give you both some quiet time in which to talk.

☙ Clean the bathroom. This might sound like a low priority, but who wants to throw up in a dirty toilet?

☙ Show interest. Yes, you're discussing baby names for the umpteenth time, but it's important to her—and ultimately to you. Go to appointments when you can; be sure to make it to the first heartbeat and the ultrasounds. Take her out to dinner. And remember to spend some time as a couple.

☙ Take childbirth classes. Don't worry about turning green or looking silly. Classes will help you tremendously once she's in labor, and will prepare you for most things along the way.

the second trimester

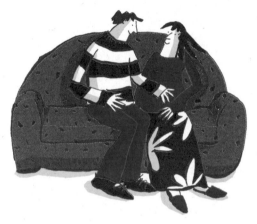

🖐 Be the one to fill the gas tank. It sounds silly, but the fumes can make her feel ill and aren't good for her or your baby.

🖐 Read a book on pregnancy. Showing her that you have your own interest in the subject may ease her fears. There are also many web sites designed for dads.

🖐 Let her nap! If she's exhausted, an hour-long nap can make a world of difference, as can sleeping in on the weekend.

🖐 Feel the baby. Try resting your hand on her belly during TV time or while you're lying in bed (ask first!).

the third trimester

Oh, you're almost there—it's so close now you can almost taste it. But while your excitement mounts, your mobility decreases and suddenly you're starting to feel as if you're walking through water wherever you go.

It's all right. You don't have to do that much now . . . except get ready for the baby, right? Not to mention that your energy is still up there, even if your ability to jump around has diminished. I know I shouldn't say it, but try to enjoy this time. It lasts for only a little while, and so many wonderful things are happening—like getting poked by baby in the ribs and bladder! No, really, it's fun to watch that belly move and respond, and soon he or she will be

the third trimester

out to harass you for real. Be patient, but be excited too, and use this time before the birth to allay your fears of labor and learn as much as you can. Talk with some moms

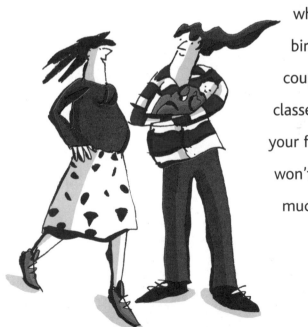

who just gave birth; take a couple more classes; and put your feet up—you won't get to for much longer.

plan early

To ease the transition to life with a baby, start planning early. Have everything in place by your 37th week, since you actually have a "due month" from 37 to 42 weeks, rather than a "due date." You will need to make a helper list, get ready for the return trip, and prepare your home (*see page 316*). To make your helper list, write down the names and phone numbers of any people whose help you might need after your baby is born: mother's caregiver (obstetrician/midwife), baby's caregiver (pediatrician/clinic), hospital nursery information line, breast-feeding counselor, La Leche League support line, public health nurse or home health agency, postpartum doula service, and so on. If you've given birth in a birth center or hospital, you'll need to take your baby home in a car seat, so install it and practice using it well before your baby arrives. You'll also need to pack a "baby" bag with clothes that are appropriate to the season for your child to wear home. Whether new or used, these clothes should be washed separately from your family's laundry with a baby-safe detergent. Pack your own going-home clothes, too. Choose loose-fitting things, as you may lose only 10–12 lb (4.5–5.5 kg) immediately after the birth.

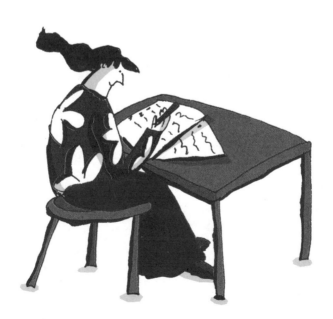

preparing your home

Plan to have your newborn sleep in your bedroom for the first few days or weeks. These steps will help you accommodate your baby:

🖐 Set up the cradle or bassinet nearby, or make your bed a safe place for your baby by removing pillows and soft bedding.

🖐 Turn a dresser into a changing table. Clear the top, and cover it with a folded towel and a changing pad. Put diaper-changing necessities on a tray. (Remember to keep one hand on your child when using this or any other elevated surface for changing.)

🖐 Add these items to keep the room clean and sanitary:

a diaper pail for soiled diapers;

a hamper for baby's laundry;

and a plastic-lined

wastebasket for

discarded cotton

balls and wipes.

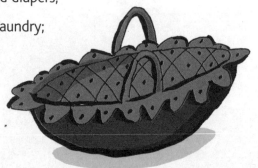

the third trimester

fear of waters breaking in public

Television programs often show the pregnant character's waters breaking—always in the middle of a restaurant (usually during a robbery or a fierce argument). Believe it or not, only 5 percent of pregnant women experience their waters breaking naturally. In most cases labor starts and, once contractions are five minutes apart and you reach the hospital, the amniotic sac is punctured manually by a nurse to progress labor. It's a painless process, and nothing to be concerned about. If by chance you are one of the few who experience water breakage naturally, you need to go to the emergency room immediately, even if your contractions have not started, because once the amniotic sac has ruptured, there is a risk of infection. Doctors usually try and deliver a baby within 24 hours of the waters breaking, so at least you have that off your mind!

braxton hicks contractions

Braxton Hicks contractions can shock the heck out of you. You'll be walking around and, all of a sudden, your belly will tighten and get fantastically hard. You might think—no, you *will* think—is this it? Am I in labor? Well, no. Sorry, you're not in labor; but, on the upside, your body is preparing for it. Your abdomen is tightening to get it ready for pushing. These "fake" contractions (although they don't necessarily feel fake) always start in the front and are really not noticeable as pain until much later on (or even until your second or third pregnancy). You'll get them most often when you're active, and they might even be severe enough to take your breath away for a minute, but real labor generally begins in the back, down low, then moves around to the abdomen, and it's a much crampier feeling. There is no better explanation, I think, than to say that if you lie down for a while, Braxton Hicks contractions will go away—

eventually. If you lie down for a while with real contractions, they will continue. Talk with your family and friends, though, because every woman begins a little differently. However, I promise that, when the baby is ready, you'll know it!

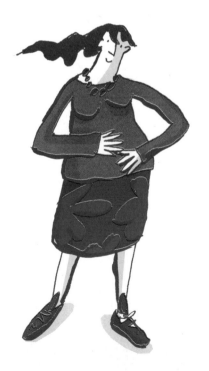

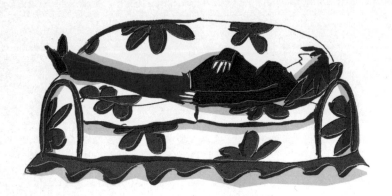

elevate your feet and legs

Just a 10–15-minute break spent lying down on your back, with both your feet and legs elevated, will do wonders for you during the third trimester, says one mom. This position will boost the circulation in your legs, help tired, achy feet, and even give your sore back a rest. This tip is great not only at the end of the day, but at any time when you can squeeze a quick rest-break in.

baby on the bladder

This is definitely one of the not-so-fun parts of pregnancy. Now that your baby is growing rapidly and is short of space, you may start to feel a sudden urge to urinate—as if your bladder is about to explode, although you can't seem to go. This is caused by the baby lying on the bladder: either resting on it or with a foot or arm pressed into it. By the time baby engages in your pelvis, you'll feel like you have to go every half hour, but this doesn't mean you should cut down on your fluid intake—you should actually be drinking more, especially in the spring and summer months. Another organ that your baby can press into is your stomach, and this can cause acid reflux (bile from the stomach passing back up the windpipe). As you get into the eighth and ninth months, your baby will increasingly seem to crush most of your organs. Don't worry—this is strictly temporary, and there isn't too much time left until your baby is born.

pelvic pressure

During your third trimester (particularly near the end), you may sometimes feel as though you are moving toward the ground—almost as if the baby is pushing you there. This pressure in your pelvic area is quite normal and usually means that the baby has "dropped"—that is, started its descent into the birth canal.

A pelvic twinge is a bit like pelvic pressure, only it can happen while you are sitting down as well as standing up, and it feels as if something is poking at your vaginal area. Even though this uncomfortable feeling may last for a minute or so, it's very common. Try to elevate your hips above your shoulders by lying on a bed or couch with some pillows under your hips. There are also "slings" on the market that strap under a woman's belly and help to support the baby. I never actually used one, but anyone who is having trouble in this area might want to investigate one of these.

balance

Balance can be difficult to manage during the last months of pregnancy. Your body is not used to your growing proportions, so you may feel as if you have equilibrium problems once in a while. During my last pregnancy (my fourth), I was woefully over-optimistic about my balancing ability. I owned a restaurant and was sure of my ability to do more than a few things at once. The upshot was that I landed on my butt at least twice, while leaping (yes, leaping) over a wet floor and one covered in flour. Fortunately, my baby was well protected (with a built-in airbag of sorts) and I was just fine.

how are you carrying?

There is an old wives' tale that says that if you're carrying high, the chances are that you're having a boy, and if you're carrying low, the chances are that you're having a girl. However, that is basically what it is—an old wives' tale—and it is not true. Each person is different when it comes to proportions, and each pregnancy is different. How your body was proportioned when you got pregnant makes a major difference to the way you'll carry. One mom says, "With my daughter I carried high, but before I had got pregnant with my son I had gained some weight, and I carried midway with him. Not to mention the fact that there is no such thing as the perfect pregnant body. Not every woman will end up having a complete, perfectly round belly when she reaches the third trimester. With my first pregnancy I had that complete round belly, but with my second pregnancy I looked a lot like I had an upper and lower belly, with kind of a small fold in between."

This is so true. In fact, I can add that with my own daughter (my second child) no one could tell I was pregnant when I sat down—even at seven months—and with my last child everyone thought I was having twins because, although from the back you couldn't tell I was pregnant, I had a huge round belly up front. Turned out he was just a healthy nine-plus-pounder!

name that body part!

This trimester is the best time to play a very entertaining game called "Name That Body Part." By now, your baby is big enough to start exploring his or her area by pressing feet, hands, and fists against your stomach. As your baby grows, he or she will press more and more body parts against your stomach—but the trick is to figure out which body part is which. Unfortunately, there isn't a surefire way of determining this, except for guessing.

You can sometimes really distinguish a foot from a hand if you press your finger across your stomach until you find a row of small bumps, which could be fingers or toes. Once you find them, slowly move the finger or palm of your hand away. If a small bulge starts to follow and run across your stomach, then the chances are it was his or her hand that you found. Next month, your baby will be a little bit bigger and will press a little harder, so you may be able to tell a bit more easily what body part is what. I used to play this neat game with my *in utero* little ones: the poking game. I would poke him or her gently in the . . . (whatever body part it was), and nine times out of ten my baby would respond with a poke or kick of his or her own. This was very effective at those times when I realized I hadn't felt any movement in a little while and I panicked!

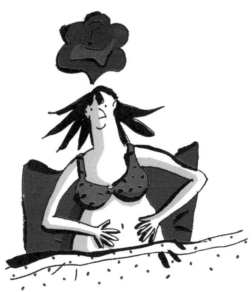

tummy-touching

I've read in many books and on many web pages about pregnant women who comment that strangers (ranging from those in the street to strangers in grocery stores and restaurants) come up and ask to touch their stomach. From what I understand, the reason people do this is because the idea of a life growing inside your stomach is fascinating to them. The thought of a stranger asking to touch your stomach may be kind of scary, but whether or not you feel comfortable with it is entirely up to you. Most women (including me) feel that a pregnant stomach is sort of a secret and personal place to be touching. So if someone you don't know asks to touch your stomach, don't be afraid to say, "No, I really don't feel comfortable with that." It's your body and it's your choice.

the nesting instinct

As your due date starts to get closer, it's very common for a pregnant woman to feel the need to clean and organize everything and anything, and make sure that all is absolutely ready for when baby comes home. This is a natural maternal instinct, and even after preparing everything, you may feel as if there is still more to do. Keep going: that extra time will vanish into thin air as soon as your baby arrives.

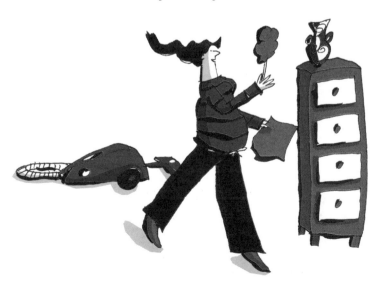

pluses and minuses

As your baby "drops" and engages in your pelvis, the pressure will be released off your lungs and you should find that you are able to breathe more easily. As baby engages, your stomach is another organ that will start to acquire more space; as a result, you will be able to hold more food and will probably feel hungrier than you have during the past few months. But if only the law of gravity could make exceptions for pregnant women! With the extra pounds of your baby and the size of your stomach, your body (and especially your legs) will not be used to handling the weight. So, instead of the normal brisk walking stride that you are used to, you'll feel as if you are waddling everywhere. And not only will the size of your stomach cause you problems with sleeping during the ninth month, but anxiety about your due day will often make it hard for you to catch a good night's sleep. It's very normal for women—especially if this is your first pregnancy—to feel anxious about labor. You will

probably be thinking: Will I know when it starts? What do I do

when it starts? How will it feel? Will I be in pain? Plus millions

of other questions and anxieties. This is totally understandable

(even if this isn't your first child), but try to concentrate on the

present, and everything else will take its course in time.

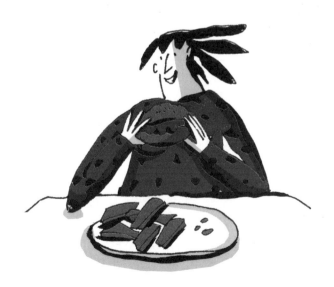

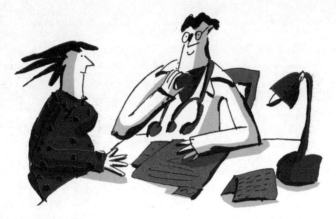

dilation

With each prenatal visit during your ninth month, your doctor will do a pelvic examination, checking at the same time to see whether or not you are dilated. Dilation occurs when the entrance to the birth canal (the cervix) starts to widen slowly so that your baby will fit through when it is time for him or her to be born. If your doctor tells you that you are 1 or 2 centimeters dilated, don't get overexcited and expect baby to be born in a few days—even if your doctor tells you that your water bag is starting to bulge through. Even if you are at 2 centimeters, it could be one to three weeks before the second stage of labor begins. Dilation is considered the first stage of labor (*see pages 368–369 for the other stages*). Dilation can be a very slow process and usually doesn't start until the second week into your ninth month. Your cervix will dilate to 10 centimeters before baby is born, and most times pain medication won't be given until you are 4 centimeters dilated. Usually by the time you are in active labor (with contractions five to eight minutes apart) and are in the hospital, you are 2 to 4 centimeters dilated and the whole process starts to go by a bit more quickly.

coloring and perming your hair

If you routinely color or perm your hair, you may find yourself wondering if it is safe to continue to do so now. Unfortunately, this isn't an easy question to answer. Both processes involve applying chemicals directly to your scalp, small amounts of which do get into your bloodstream. In animal studies, hair chemicals have been linked to birth defects, but these appear to happen only with a significantly larger exposure than you get with routine hair treatments. Most research (albeit limited) does show that it is safe to color and perm your hair while you are pregnant. Based on common sense, however, doctors often suggest waiting until after the first trimester, because this is the time when your baby's development is most influenced by outside factors. An alternative that may work for you is highlighting or frosting your hair. With these two methods, very little of the color touches your scalp, which minimizes your exposure to chemicals. Another important consideration before getting a perm is that your hair may be unpredictable in the way it reacts to treatment during pregnancy. Although many people—including hair stylists—attribute this unpredictability to the "raging hormones" of pregnancy, the bottom line is that a perm may leave your hair straight, make your hair frizz, or wave your hair in some areas, but not in others. Of course, the decision about whether or not to dye or perm your hair is up to you. Discuss with your health-care practitioner her views about hair chemicals to help you make your decision.

massages

Many pregnant women find that a massage is an excellent way to rejuvenate themselves and relax. After 20 or so weeks of pregnancy, however, it's important to remember not to lie flat on your back. A large vessel to your heart (called the vena cava) lies along the back wall of your abdomen, next to your spine, and can be compressed by the weight of your uterus when you lie flat on your back. Instead, get the person giving you the massage to prop a pillow under your right hip when you lie down. This tips the uterus off the major blood vessels. Many massage therapists offer a table made especially for pregnant women, with a cutout in the middle for your pregnant belly, and you may find this position much more comfortable when having your back massaged. If your masseuse does not have this type of table, it is best not to lie fully on your stomach (for obvious reasons, not the least of which is your own discomfort). Instead, lie on your side for this portion of the massage. If she massages your abdomen, be careful that it does not cause you to have contractions—if you do experience any, stop this part of the massage.

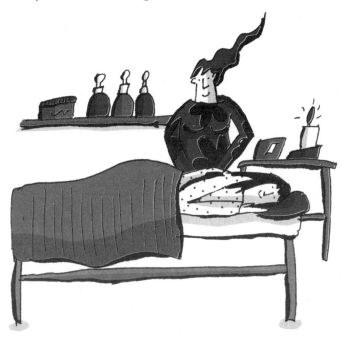

fingers and toes

During pregnancy, you may be pleasantly surprised to find your fingernails and toenails growing faster and stronger than usual. If you choose to get a pedicure, you will also be taking care of the increasingly difficult task of cutting your toenails as your belly begins to interfere with your ability to reach your own feet! Try to ensure that you sit in an area of the salon with plenty of ventilation, so that you are not exposed to any fumes from products such as nail polish for a long period of time.

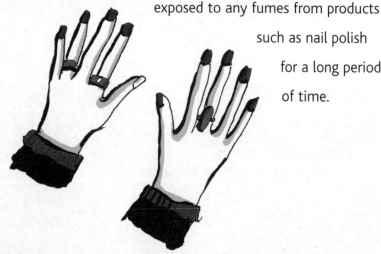

doulas

A doula is a woman trained in the emotional and physical support of women in labor, and is usually hired by the family to be an extra support person for the woman and her partner. Some doulas are certified by the organization Doulas of North America (DONA, see *www.dona.org*). Most doulas will meet the family before the birth, talk about the birth plan, and then support the family through labor and birth—and sometimes beyond. Doulas do not provide medical care to women in labor, and do not deliver babies. Studies have shown that women attended by doulas have lower cesarean rates and use fewer epidurals than those with traditional labor support. Doulas do not undercut fathers during delivery: A study of the involvement of the father in doula-supported labors showed the same (or more) contact between the father and mother, compared with when the father was the only coach.

pack a bag

Pack a bag for the hospital before you go into labor, since throwing things into a suitcase is not something you want to do when you're in the midst of painful contractions. Don't fret about what to take with you: here's a handy list of things you might want to remember. You may not end up using all of these items, but better to have them with you during labor than to regret what you left at home:

- Insurance card or hospital registration papers
- Favorite pillow
- Special picture or object that you have chosen as your focal point
- Bathrobe
- Slippers (for walking the halls as your labor progresses)
- Socks

the third trimester

- Lollipops (to keep your mouth moist)
- Lip balm (the dry air in the hospital, as well as breathing exercises, can take a toll on your lips)
- Toothbrush and toothpaste (refreshing to use during labor)
- CD or tape player and your favorite relaxing music
- Lotion or oil (for your coach's massages)
- Tennis ball (for your coach to rub on your lower back as counterpressure)
- Barrette or hair band
- Glasses, if you wear them (some hospitals don't allow patients to wear contact lenses while in labor)
- Camera with extra rolls of film and extra batteries
- Video camera
- Phone list of friends and relatives
- Baby book (if you want to have your baby's footprints taken).

timely questions

Many times, procedures are recommended in situations that require fast action for medical reasons. When decisions need to be made quickly, it may be hard to think of all the questions you need to ask to make an informed choice. Here is a list to prompt you to think of points that you may want to discuss with your practitioner in these situations. You might want to write this list out or photocopy it and keep it handy:

- What is my particular problem?
- Why is it a problem?
- How serious is it?
- Can you describe the suggested treatment?
- Why is it necessary (i.e., how will it benefit me or the baby)?
- What are the risks?
- Will the treatment resolve my problem completely or simply alleviate it?

🖐 If this doesn't succeed, what will we do next?

🖐 Why does it need to be done now? What happens if we wait
   a little longer to do it?

🖐 What happens if we decide not to do it?

🖐 What other alternatives are there?

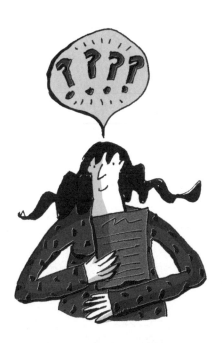

address your fears

Most women (and men) have some element of fear as they approach labor and delivery. When should we go to the hospital? What exactly is an episiotomy? Do I have to be connected to the fetal monitor throughout my labor? How much pain will there be? Knowledge may not quell all anxieties, but it will help you feel more prepared to meet the challenge of childbirth together.

Learn techniques to deal with pain: classes teach you different methods of achieving this. These may well include breathing and relaxation exercises, visualization, and other comforting activities.

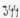

classes to take

Check with your hospital or childbirth association for classes
that you and your family can attend, including the following:

🖐 Early pregnancy classes

🖐 Cesarean birth classes

🖐 VBAC (Vaginal Birth After Cesarean) classes

🖐 Breast-feeding classes

🖐 Infant-care basics classes

🖐 Infant and child
cardiopulmonary
resuscitation (CPR,
or mouth-to-mouth
resuscitation) classes

🖐 Baby-massage classes

🖐 Sibling classes

🖐 Grandparent classes.

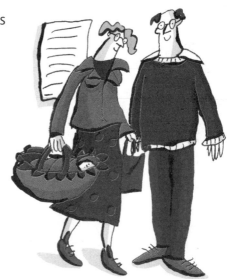

plan the birth

In addition to preparing for labor through childbirth education and practicing relaxation techniques, what can you do to get the experience you want? Although luck always plays a part in the way your labor goes, you can take some action to help yourself have a low-tech experience, if that is what you want. In some hospitals today, more than 70 percent of mothers are given an epidural, so if you are seeking an unmedicated birth experience, it may help to plan ahead and write down your birth plan (*see page 348*). Other tips:

🖐 Pick your practitioner carefully. Be sure that you have chosen a practitioner who can support your specific desires.

🖐 Consider getting extra labor support. In addition to your partner, think about inviting along a female friend or relative who has had a natural childbirth, or hiring a doula (*see page 339*) to help you through. Although your partner is the one who cares about you most, and knows you best, most fathers are not ready to be the sole coach for a mother in labor. It is distressing to see your loved one in pain, and hard to keep a perspective on how close the finish line is. In addition, there is a lot to know about comfort measures during labor, and not all fathers spend the necessary time preparing for the role of coach.

Make your wishes known ahead of time. Communicate in advance what you want out of the experience. You will not be thinking clearly in labor, and will find it hard to make decisions, so tell your team if you don't want pain medication offered to you, and instruct them ahead of time on what you want them to do if you ask. Because many women will ask for medication anyway during the stress of the transition phase of labor, consider agreeing on a code word that is a sure indication that you are really changing your mind.

write down your birth plan

Instead of writing a traditional bullet-point list, you might want to write your birth plan as a letter, explaining the sort of experience that you are seeking. If you can keep it short and focus on your priorities, it will be easier for your practitioner to read, and less overwhelming. Be sure to say clearly that you trust the hospital team to do the right thing for you and your baby, and to make some decisions for you in the case of an emergency. Communicate with your team: talk again to your doctor or midwife about what you are seeking. Ask her how realistic she thinks your goals are, given the location where you will deliver and how your pregnancy has been progressing. Not surprisingly, many practitioners aren't comfortable signing a birth plan as if it were a contract. Even if they support all your wishes, they can't promise that things will go as you want them to.

think natural first

Some labors are more "doable" than others. One option, if you can't decide what type of childbirth you want, is to prepare for natural childbirth and see what happens. You can change the plan if you have a long labor or get exhausted. Intravenous pain medicine such as Nubain or Demerol can take the edge off contractions, if you want some help but don't need an epidural. These medications interfere less with the progress of labor.

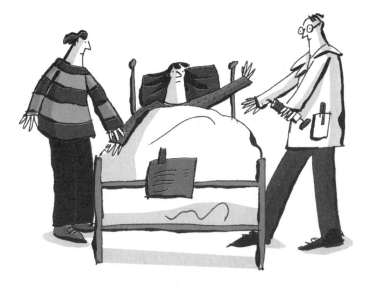

methods of prepared childbirth

There are three main methods of prepared childbirth. Many
instructors include elements from each, plus guided imagery,
music therapy, and other relaxation techniques. Contact your
practitioner's office, your hospital, or your area childbirth
education association for further information.

The Dick-Read method dates back to the 1940s, and was
one of the first organized approaches to childbirth education.
It assumes that lack of knowledge (or incorrect knowledge)
about childbirth leads to fear; this fear causes tension, which
then contributes to increased pain. So understanding how labor
affects different parts of the body can help to do away with fear.

The Lamaze method, named for Dr. Fernand Lamaze, prepares
women to deal actively with contractions. Each woman is
conditioned (trained) to respond to her contractions with
relaxation, while breathing exercises act as a distraction from

the discomfort. This method integrates the father as a coach and encourages couples to share in the birth of their child. It is one of the more popular approaches to managing the pain of labor.

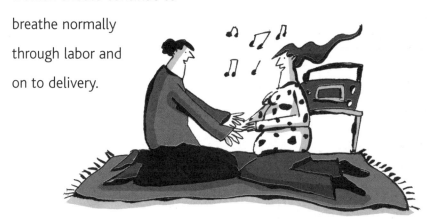 Dr. Robert Bradley's method emphasizes the father's role as coach, based on the belief that his active participation is vital to the childbirth experience. Couples often attend classes much earlier on in the pregnancy, and Dr. Bradley believes that a woman should continue to breathe normally through labor and on to delivery.

getting ready to breast-feed

Laura Jana, M.D., says, "Women with any size or shape of breasts can successfully breast-feed. During your pregnancy, your breasts will undergo certain changes whether or not you intend to breast-feed. Some women experience a period of breast tenderness, and many notice breast enlargement. Toward the end of your pregnancy, you may experience some leakage of colostrum [a practice milk that is rich in protein]. There are several things you can do to prepare yourself and your body for these changes and for breast-feeding when your baby is born."

Create a supportive environment. Be sure that the obstetrician, pediatrician, nurse practitioner, or family practitioner you choose is supportive of, and enthusiastic about, your decision to breast-feed and will be able to answer all your questions. Educate yourself; breast-feeding is supposed to be one of the most natural things a mother can do, but that doesn't mean it always comes naturally. Any woman planning to breast-feed for the first time can benefit from reading about the subject, taking birthing classes that teach breast-feeding techniques, and making sure she will deliver in a supportive environment. And prepare yourself physically. Should you toughen your nipples? Although several regimens used to be recommended to toughen the nipples in preparation for nursing, many experts now agree that this is not necessary to prevent soreness once you begin breast-feeding. Avoid the use of soaps and other irritating or drying agents on your nipples during pregnancy and while you are nursing.

breast-feeding support

Some women have nipples that do not stick out, or that pull in at the center, even when stimulated. Women with flat or inverted nipples can often breast-feed successfully even if nothing is done about them during pregnancy. However, there are some simple interventions—including the use of breast shields or a simple massage technique (known as the Hoffman Technique)—that can help to prevent unnecessary frustration with breast-feeding when the baby is born. If you suspect that you have inverted nipples, check with your health-care provider or contact a lactation resource such as La Leche League for advice. If your breasts enlarge during pregnancy, do not hesitate to buy bras with larger cup sizes. Remember that comfort is as important as support, and be aware that your breast size may continue to increase once your baby is born and you begin nursing. For this reason, limit the number of nursing bras that you buy toward the end of your pregnancy to just two or three, until you have begun breast-feeding and have determined which bra size is most comfortable for you.

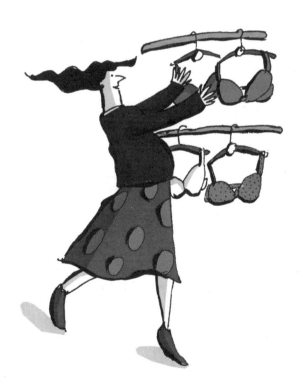

the third trimester

get things clear in your mind

Here are some steps to getting the birth experience you want:

👋 Have a clear sense in your own mind of the kind of experience you seek. Are you leaning toward natural childbirth? Do you want to have an epidural? Do you want to feel that you are being monitored medically for problems, or allowed to be on your own more? These leanings can help you decide on your practitioner and the place in which to give birth—and these decisions may have more effect on your experience than any "birth plan" that you create. Note that many practitioners deliver at only one or two locations, so these two decisions are closely related.

👋 Educate yourself, for there are many ways to have a baby. Learn about labor and birth and all of your options in greater detail. Read, talk to friends, and choose a childbirth preparation method that reflects your own philosophy.

the third trimester

✋ Get a feel for what it's like to have a baby at the site you have chosen. Many hospitals provide tours of their labor and delivery units. Find out about routine procedures and policies of the birthing unit and of your OB's (obstetrician's) practice group.

✋ Ask questions, and check with your practitioner and with friends who have delivered there. For example, some hospitals have a limit on the number of people who can be with you in labor, or a policy on videotaping deliveries; some units have birthing tubs or showers in the rooms to help you relax. Understanding these issues can help you to appreciate the choices that are open to you.

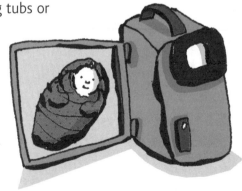

go with your instincts

I had an interesting range of experiences in birthing my four children. My first one was a standard hospital birth attended by obstetricians, and the experience was—well, I'll be honest—horrible. I had no idea that midwives and certified nurse-midwives were a viable option for a healthy delivery. My next birth was a wonderful experience in a hospital, but with an understanding midwife who let me birth on the floor of my room (over a sheet) and caught my daughter—quite literally—as she came out fast. My third birth was a home birth, attended by a wonderful nurse-midwife and a local EMT (just in case). I took the precaution of donating some money to the local volunteer fire department/ambulance service and letting them know my due date, so they would be on alert! I also rented an oxygen tank and other equipment recommended by my midwife. Fortunately, none of it was necessary and I labored, delivered, and recovered on the couch in my living room. For my fourth birth, I headed back to the hospital; although I found the home birth wonderful, it was a bit more stressful because I worried about "entertaining" my midwife and keeping the house clean. Armed with much experience and three natural births, I had no problems delivering at an Ivy League teaching hospital with a midwife and a medical student experiencing her first birth. And the point of telling you all this? Each birth is different and each woman is different. The key is finding what is right for you and your baby, and not worrying about what your friend, your mother, or I did when having our babies. If obstetricians and hospitals make you feel comfortable—then go to one. But don't be pushed into it if you'd rather try a more relaxed environment. This is *your* birth experience, and in the end you have to push that little one out!

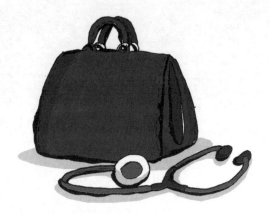

birthing places

Here is a description of the wide range of birthing places on offer:

In the U.S., most babies are born in hospital. Teaching hospitals generally have the greatest availability of specialists and high-tech medical treatments, but will often get more people (including trainees such as residents and students) involved in your care.

Community hospitals often have higher cesarean rates than teaching hospitals. Obstetricians, family doctors, and nurse-midwives can all deliver babies in a community hospital.

the third trimester

Individual hospitals differ in their epidural and cesarean rates and their availability of anesthesia and emergency consultation. Many hospitals now have low-tech labor/delivery/recovery rooms for uncomplicated births, as well as delivery-operating rooms for when the needs are more medical. Ask your practitioner about the settings in which he or she delivers.

Birth centers may be independent or attached to a hospital. They offer a more homelike environment than hospitals, and usually provide only for natural, unmedicated childbirth (and have a low rate of cesarean section). If a complication arises, the woman or the newborn may be transferred to hospital.

Home birth is not a common choice in the U.S. today. Most obstetricians (and many parents) believe that childbirth at home is not safe. If you are considering a home birth, be sure to educate yourself about the risks, as well as potential benefits.

It Worked For Me . . .

labor and delivery

What can I say? It's a little scary and a lot exciting.
It also encompasses a million other emotions, ranging
from elation to exhaustion. There will be many times
before you're actually in labor when you'll feel a twinge or
a contraction and wonder, "Is this it?" Your heart will beat
faster and your stomach will turn over a bit . . . only for
you to realize that the contraction has gone away.

You may feel disappointed or relieved. But soon it
will be for real, and all of a sudden your wish that it would
"hurry up and be over with" will go out the window and
you may find yourself thinking, "Wait, give me a minute!"
Take a breath. Take two, and prepare to give birth.

labor and delivery

The following section offers lots of tips to help you. You won't remember them all—but if you can remember only one to get you through labor and delivery, it should be this: just breathe, in and out, in and out (*see pages 388–389*). It doesn't have to be Lamaze-style breathing exercises, but breathe and know that your baby is coming out one way or another—and yes, you can do it—and it will be amazing when the new arrival is finally here.

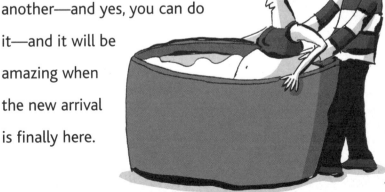

warning signs of labor

After the eighth month of pregnancy, time seems to pass slowly. As your belly gets bigger, your patience gets shorter and you can't wait to give birth. For first-time moms, this can be a scary experience because you don't know what to expect. Labor is when your cervix begins to dilate and becomes thinner, making room for your baby to pass through. The following questions will help you know if you are going into labor:

❀ Have people begun telling you that you have dropped or lightened? This is when the baby positions himself or herself for birth. You will notice that you can breathe normally again.

❀ Take a walk: do you feel that the contractions are getting stronger? This is a sign that you are in labor. If your contractions become weaker, it is a sign of false labor.

❀ Have you had a "bloody show"? This is when the mucus plug sealing the entrance to the cervix falls out. It looks like a blob of jelly with some blood in it, and is a sign that the baby is coming.

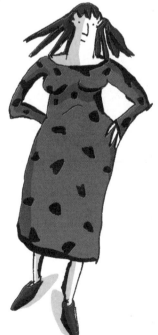 Have your waters broken? This is when a clear, odorless liquid rushes or oozes out of your vagina. Get ready: this is a sign that the contractions will become stronger and closer within 6 to 12 hours.

 Are you having back pain? As your contractions become stronger, you may start feeling them in your back.

 Do you have a compulsive urge to clean? This is known as "nesting" and is a sign that you are closer to labor.

 Has your constipation gone away? Or have you developed diarrhea? This empties your bowel to make more room for your baby.

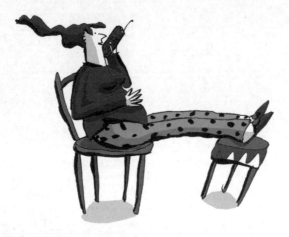

first stage: latent phase

The first stage of labor begins with the onset of regular

contractions and ends when your cervix is completely dilated; it is

broken down into three phases. (The second and third stages occur

when you have to squeeze the baby out, and when the placenta is

expelled.) The latent phase is the longest of the three, helping the

cervix to dilate up to three or four centimeters as it "effaces," or

softens and thins out. This can take five hours or more, and

labor and delivery

dilation may seem to move along slowly for many hours. Your contractions will last for about 30–40 seconds during this phase, with the interval between them shortening to about five minutes apart. Typically, these contractions are mild and easy to manage— some women describe them as similar to menstrual cramps. You will feel contractions in the lower back and toward the front of your lower abdomen. Many women have mixed emotions during this phase. They can be excited and happy, knowing that the end of pregnancy is near. They also may feel some apprehension— especially first-time moms. Although you may have a lot of energy at this time, you should eat lightly, drink to satisfy your thirst, and rest. Conserving energy is the name of the game, for labor may continue longer than anticipated. This is the time to alert those who make up your support team, so get on the phone to them and tell them to stand by, ready to accompany you to the hospital.

middle phase

During the middle (or active) phase of first-stage labor, your cervix dilates at an accelerated rate to about seven centimeters. This phase usually lasts for around three hours, with your contractions becoming more intense and regular, three to five minutes apart and lasting for about 60 seconds. At this time, you need to increase your concentration during contractions, which may be feeling more painful. Some women request drugs now. A "bloody show" (*see pages 364–365*) can occur, with mucus that is bloodier than the pinkish-tinged mucus of early labor, but this is not a cause for alarm. However, as this phase progresses, you may feel less talkative, for your focus will become more inward. If you are not tired, you can sit up or walk around and you should try to change positions often—at least every 30 minutes. In some facilities, you may be able to shower or relax in a warm tub. It's essential that you get supportive coaching and relaxation now.

transition phase

This phase involves the final stretching of your cervix before your baby moves down into the birth canal. It is a short but increasingly intense phase, usually lasting for about two hours, when your cervix dilates from 8 to 10 centimeters. Your contractions will become very powerful, two to three minutes apart and lasting for 60–90 seconds, allowing you little rest between them. At this point, you must concentrate on working with your breathing and your body's natural rhythm, and you may need some direct coaching. Some moms say they became irritable and sensitive to their environment at this time; other women experienced trembling, hot and cold flashes, nausea, vomiting, and mercurial emotions. If your bag of waters has not already broken, it probably will during transition. You may also experience the urge to push as your baby travels downward into the birth canal.

should I stay or should I go?

If you are less than 35 weeks pregnant and you have regular contractions lasting more than 30 seconds and occurring more than four to six times an hour, try resting and drinking lots of fluids. If the contractions don't settle down with these changes in activity, call your practitioner. The signs of preterm labor can be subtle and should be evaluated.

Once you are past 36 weeks, and if this is a first pregnancy, you are much more likely to go to your birth place too early than too late. Don't time contractions until they are painful and regular. Plan to go to the hospital when they are so strong that you cannot hold a conversation during one; they are closer than five minutes apart; and they continue in that pattern for more than an hour. For women who have given birth before, Marjorie Greenfield, M.D., recommends using your previous labor as a guideline. On average, second babies come in half the time it took for the first. Subsequent pregnancies are usually similar to the second one. If you just aren't sure whether it is false or real labor, don't feel bad about going into the labor and delivery ward to be examined. Your practitioner and the nurses there see many women in false labor each day. And sometimes it is hard even for the professionals to tell whether it is the real thing.

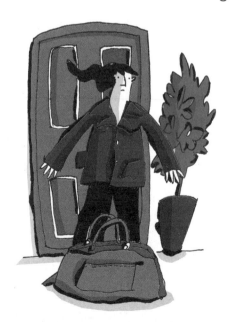

natural ways to induce labor

As you near the end of your pregnancy, you may be ready for the entire process of carrying your baby to be over. You might wonder: is it safe to try to naturally induce labor, and how do I set about accomplishing this? You shouldn't even consider this until you are around 40 weeks pregnant, or overdue. That's because your due date could be inaccurate by a few weeks, and if you start labor before 40 weeks you might give birth to the baby before he or she is ready to thrive outside the womb.

Several measures might make you have contractions and start labor, but they'll work only if your body is ready; if it isn't, you will only frustrate yourself. Use caution when trying any of these natural methods to begin labor, particularly herbs and nipple stimulation, and make sure you discuss them with your practitioner before trying them. To be successful, most of them require you to be having contractions or in early labor.

labor and delivery

✋ Walk: if you are having contractions but are not yet in labor, walking can help get things going. It allows your hips to sway from side to side, which will help bring the baby into the correct position to be born. And by standing upright you're using gravity to move the baby down into the pelvis.

✋ Sex: making love may be one of the last things on your mind, but believe it or not, sex is one of the best things you can do to get labor under way. When you and your partner make love, his semen (which contains prostaglandins) and your orgasm (which produces oxytocin) can stimulate contractions. A double dose—a few hours apart—might give you even better results.

more ways to encourage labor

👋 Blue and black cohosh: These herbs are often used to induce labor and may be particularly helpful if you are having weak or irregular contractions. Blue cohosh is believed to make uterine contractions stronger; black cohosh to regulate contractions. Unfortunately no studies have determined that these natural treatments are safe, or whether all versions of the herb are of equal potency. Be sure to discuss any herbal treatment with your medical practitioner to establish if it is a good idea for you.

👋 Nipple stimulation: some women massage their nipples as a way to induce labor. This brings about the release of oxytocin, which causes contractions and may evolve into labor. Most practitioners are not enthusiastic about this method, because it has been known to lead to excessively long, strong uterine contractions and fetal distress. Unless your practitioner advises it, this is not recommended as a means of beginning labor.

labor and delivery

🖐 Castor oil: for decades, women have used castor oil to help induce labor, and it can give good results if you are in early labor. It is believed to work by causing spasms in the intestines, which in turn cause the uterus to cramp. You can take 1–2 fl oz (30–60 ml) castor oil mixed with 6 fl oz (175 ml) orange juice to cut its oiliness. Some practitioners suggest taking a single dose; others repeated doses, but always check with them first. Keep in mind that castor oil will usually cause your bowels to empty within about three hours.

🖐 Spicy food: some people swear it was that extra-hot enchilada that brought them face to face with their baby. You could try it, but if you have a full stomach in labor, you are more likely to be nauseated or to vomit.

stripping the membranes

Your practitioner may offer to "strip your membranes" to help start your labor. This procedure usually feels like a vaginal examination, although some moms find it painful or that it causes cramping. The practitioner places her gloved finger through your cervix and sweeps the amniotic membranes free of their attachment to the lower part of the uterine cavity. This is believed to release hormonelike substances called prostaglandins, which help to ready your body for labor. Although some experts believe that stripping the membranes causes you to go into labor that day, the only research was done by a group of midwives who stripped the membranes of a number of their patients at every visit after 38 weeks' gestation. Their findings showed that patients who had this procedure were less likely to go past their due dates; the process didn't seem to pose any complications or cause the patients' waters to break.

artificial induction

If you have gone beyond 42 weeks, suffer from pre-eclampsia, kidney disease, or diabetes, or your pediatrician believes that your baby's well-being may be suffering, then he or she may have to be induced (meaning that your labor is started by artificial means). If you consent to being induced, refuse to allow your bag of waters to be broken before you are established in active, progressive labor. Once the membranes are ruptured, you are committed to delivery, which will be by cesarean if the induction doesn't "take." Artificial methods of induction include rupturing the membranes, inserting a gel or suppository into the vagina to ripen the cervix, inserting a Foley catheter into the cervix, and using Pitocin intravenously to start your contractions.

tips for coaches

The following tips should enable your birth coach to be in the best position to assist you as you enter the second stage of labor:

🖐 Be prepared. You should attend birthing classes with the mom-to-be before the due date. You will learn many techniques that will help you cope when the big day arrives.

🖐 Know what to expect. It is a good idea to go on a tour of the hospital to get familiar with its layout. Talk to nurses or other staff members to get an idea of what will happen on delivery day and what you should expect.

🖐 Be patient. The process of labor and delivery is often lengthy; that's why it's important to be ready to wait.

🖐 Be supportive. She will need you there to be her advocate and cheerleader. Take time to comfort and distract her with warm showers or by rubbing her lower back.

🖐 Bring along items for yourself. You may be at the hospital for

labor and delivery

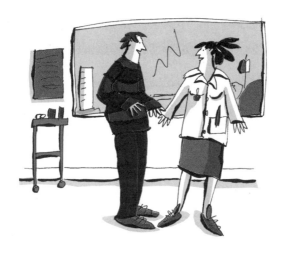

many hours, so it is important to bring with you the things you may need, like a bathing suit (so that you can take warm showers with the mom), snacks, comfortable shoes for walking up and down the hallways, toiletries, and a change of clothes.

Make decisions. At times, you will have to evaluate the situation and act quickly, based on the information you have. For example, if the mom is in severe pain and wants an epidural, you may have to find a nurse or doctor who will be able to help.

more tips for coaches

Know her expectations. You and the mom should discuss your joint expectations for the day of delivery. It is critical to know what she wants, and expects, before arriving at the hospital. For instance, does she want to use breathing techniques? Does she want the midwife to play a critical role? Does she want you to be hands-on? A written birth plan (*see page 348*) will help clarify these points. Of course, when the contractions are in high gear, many of these decisions may go out the window! That's okay, too. During

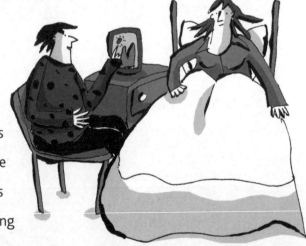

labor and delivery

labor, the mom will generally do anything that helps her get through it, which may include abandoning her birth plan.

🖐 Find a distraction. As the contraction pains begin to get closer and more painful, it is recommended that you and the mom find a distraction that will take her mind off what's happening. Some people bring items from home, like a photo or teddy bear that the mom can focus on. Others find distractions in the hospital room, like a spot on the wall or on the ceiling.

🖐 Be flexible and understanding. Mom will get so focused during the contractions that she may not want or need you after all. She may seem to ignore you, or get angry at you or others in the room. Remember not to take anything said during labor personally. She will miraculously change when the baby is born!

🖐 Remember, just having you there will mean so much to her. You will be there every step of this emotional journey!

hints on getting through labor

No one will tell you that labor is going to be easy. But through a well-organized childbirth class you can learn strategies that will help you through the final push into parenthood. Here are a few other ideas that may be helpful:

🖐 Create a peaceful and soothing environment by dimming the lights. Bring an extra pillow or cushion. If there is something else special you want to bring, call the hospital to ask if it's okay.

🖐 Have your labor coach give you lots of massages, especially on your lower back and feet.

🖐 Bring a cassette or CD player with your favorite music.

🖐 Take a warm bath or shower in your birthing room.

🖐 If heat doesn't work, try cool compresses on your lower back and forehead.

🖐 Don't be afraid to make a lot of noise: moan and groan when a contraction happens.

labor and delivery

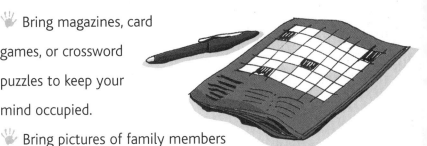

🖐 Bring magazines, card games, or crossword puzzles to keep your mind occupied.

🖐 Bring pictures of family members and place them on your nightstand. You can look at them as you lie in bed.

🖐 Try to keep moving by taking long walks up and down the hallways or by dancing with your partner.

🖐 Remember the tips you were taught in your childbirth class. Keep breathing, visualizing, and looking to your labor coach for constant companionship.

🖐 Try different positions: sitting or standing, squatting, lying on your side, crouching on your hands and knees—even sitting on the toilet. Find whatever pose helps you through the contractions.

relaxation strategies

These strategies come from Martha Sears, R.N. and wife of famous pediatrician William Sears (she is also the mother of their eight children).

To practice relaxation with your partner, you need to be very comfortable. Collect a bunch of pillows and tell your partner where you like them. Do these exercises in various positions: standing and leaning against your partner, a wall, or a piece of furniture; sitting down; lying on your side; and even on all fours.

Check your whole body for muscle tension: a furrowed forehead, clenched fists, and a tight mouth are the easiest ones to spot. Then practice systematically releasing each group of muscles from head to toe. Tense and then relax each muscle group to help you identify the two different states. When your partner cues you with "Contraction," think, "Relax and release." Then feel these tight muscles loosen.

Practice touch relaxation. This conditions you to expect pleasure rather than pain to follow tension. Find out which touches, and what kind of massage, relax you best. Follow the same head-to-toe progression as described above. Tense each muscle group and then have your partner apply a warm, relaxed touch to that area as your cue to release the tension. This means you don't have to keep hearing the verbal cue "Relax," which eventually becomes irritating. Another goal is to be able to relax a tense muscle when your partner puts just the right touch on that spot before it begins to hurt. Practice: "I hurt here— you press hard [or stroke or touch] here."

the power of visualization

Use visualization to help you relax: a clear mind filled with soothing scenes soothes a laboring body—at least between contractions. It also encourages the production of labor-enhancing endorphins. Sports psychologists use mental imagery or visualization to help athletes perform. Follow these steps to use visualization for relaxation during labor:

🖐 Determine the scenes that you find most relaxing (rolling waves, waterfalls, meandering streams, walking along the beach with your mate) and practice meditating on them often throughout the day, especially in the final month of pregnancy.

🖐 Think about appropriate images to use during contractions. When a contraction begins, picture your uterus "hugging" your baby and pulling itself up over his or her adorable little head. During the dilating stage, imagine your cervix getting thinner and more open with each contraction.

labor and delivery

🖐 Change scenes from painful to pleasant. Grab the pain as if it were a big glob of modeling clay, massage it into a tiny ball, wrap it up, put it in a helium balloon, and imagine it leaving your body and floating up into the sky.

🖐 Between and during the more painful contractions, imagine the prize rather than the pain you have to go through to get it. Picture yourself reaching down as your baby comes out, assisting your birth attendant in placing your baby on your abdomen, and nestling your child against your breasts.

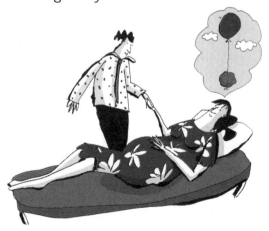

just breathe

Breathe naturally between contractions, as you do when you are falling asleep. When a contraction begins, inhale deeply and slowly through your nose, then exhale slowly through your mouth in a long, steady stream. As you breathe out, let your facial muscles relax and your limbs go limp: think of this exhalation as a long 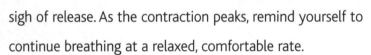 sigh of release. As the contraction peaks, remind yourself to continue breathing at a relaxed, comfortable rate.

Ask your partner to tell you to slow down if you start breathing too fast in response to an intense contraction. Have him take slow, relaxed breaths with you. If you still find yourself breathing too fast, stop for a minute and take a deep breath, followed by a long, drawn-out blow, as if you are blowing off steam. Do this periodically to remind yourself to slow down. Partners should watch your breathing patterns for cues as to how you are coping. Slow, deep, rhythmic breathing shows that you are handling your contractions well. Fast, spasmodic breathing communicates tension and anxiety.

Don't pant, however often you've seen it in the movies! Panting is not natural for humans: it exhausts you, lessens your oxygen intake, and may lead to hyperventilation, which blows off too much carbon dioxide, causing you to feel light-headed and get tingling sensations in your fingers, toes, and face. If you start to hyperventilate, breathe in through your nose and out through your mouth, as slowly as you can. And don't hold your breath. Even during the strain of pushing, the blue-in-the-face breath-holding you see in movies is not only exhausting but deprives you and your baby of much-needed oxygen.

a bag of tricks

🖐 Bring music to birth by. Studies show that moms who use music during labor require fewer pain-relieving drugs than those who do not, because music stimulates your body to release natural pain-relieving hormones. Play a medley of favorites, taking care to choose songs whose rhythms relax you rather than rev you up; bring along a player, and fresh batteries, too.

🖐 Sit on a birth ball. This is a 28-inch (70-cm) physiotherapy ball, which naturally relaxes the pelvic muscles when you sit on it.

🖐 Bring along pillows and foam wedges. You will need at least four. Thick, tapered foam wedges make relaxing back supports for sitting; a thinner one can be used as a cushion between the bed and your abdomen when you're lying on your side.

🖐 Try hot and cold packs. Hot packs improve blood flow to the tissues; cold packs lessen pain perception. A hot water bottle, or a rubber surgical glove filled with warm water, makes a fine hot

labor and delivery

pack to nestle against your lower abdomen, groin, or thigh to relieve achy muscles, or just to relax you. Packs of frozen veggies, covered with a cloth, work well as cold packs to soothe a hot forehead or numb an aching back.

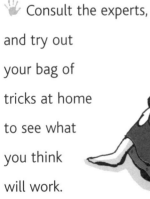 Try a beanbag chair. When you shop, try out various beanbag chairs until you find a squishy nest that you can imagine yourself sinking into during early labor. (But never put a baby in a beanbag chair.)

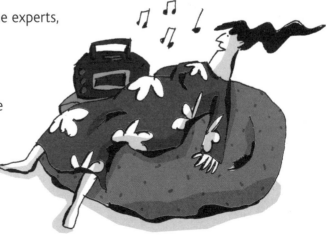 Consult the experts, and try out your bag of tricks at home to see what you think will work.

electronic fetal monitoring

Electronic fetal monitoring (EFM) is a controversial procedure because it "medicalizes" the natural birth process. You may find a midwife against it and a doctor all for it—or vice versa, depending on the circumstances. The point of EFM is to detect complications during labor, such as hypoxia (lack of oxygen to the baby) and metabolic acidosis (which can cause brain damage and/or cerebral palsy). Although cesarean section rates have actually increased since the technology was introduced in the 1950s, the number of stillbirths has been reduced to almost nothing and most doctors (and nurses) would say that EFM is an accurate way of finding out how your baby is doing during labor.

There are two types of EFM: internal and external. Internal, from what I've been told, is more painful during labor and is rarely used except when readings on an external monitor are erratic. The external monitor can be painful, too, as your contracting belly tightens the belt. The monitor may reduce your stress about the baby's condition, but let me add that if you have had a healthy pregnancy and are having a normal labor, don't feel the need to rely exclusively on this technology and relegate yourself to bed. Let your care provider know that you intend to get up and walk around—as I did during my second hospital birth.

There are several good reasons to rely on EFM: a vaginal birth after a cesarean, any high-risk pregnancy (those with diabetes, hypertension, or other complications), an inability to detect the fetal heartbeat, or a difficult labor. EFM is routinely done in hospitals, but is not essential in most cases. Speak your mind if you would rather not have it done. Monitors are restrictive and, as I said before, they can be painful, although they can also be reassuring and kind of "neat" for a first birth.

the pain of labor

What will it be like? Will I be able to handle it? The answers:
"Very painful," and "Yes, absolutely."

   As the veteran of four natural childbirths of varying intensity
and length, I can confirm that it can be done without drugs or
other therapies. I can also tell you that breathing techniques
worked not one bit for me, although some women swear by them.
You just have to decide for yourself if you want to be drug-free
sufficiently badly to go through with it. With my first child,
I was steadfast: I refused drugs right and left, but then it got to a
point where I said to myself, "Oh, my God, if it gets worse than
this, I'm going to die." I can vividly remember that moment, and
then I begged for the anesthesiologist. Turned out that I was in
transition and ready to push my extremely large-headed son
out—and an epidural was no longer an option. There are times,
however, when a woman has been laboring for so long that she's

labor and delivery

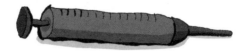

tired and can't deal mentally with the strain anymore, or maybe just doesn't want to, and then drugs are an option. Systemic painkillers such as narcotics or tranquilizers will dull pain, but not eliminate it. They are given through an IV line or injected, and will affect your entire body, not just the pelvic area (like an epidural). They'll make you sleepy, but not unconscious. This type of medication can help a woman who is "stressing" to relax a little and concentrate on pushing her baby out. It is also easier to give than an epidural into the spine. However, side effects such as dizziness, disorientation, and nausea are relatively common, and, if given too early in labor, narcotics can slow your progress; they also cross the placenta and may make your baby sleepier, affecting the ability to nurse and bond with you right after the birth. In rare cases, narcotics can make it harder for your baby to breathe.

epidural

An epidural is a regional anesthetic that decreases the feeling in the lower area of your body while you remain fully conscious. It is delivered by catheter just outside the membrane that surrounds your spine, after an anesthesiologist has injected a needle into your lower back. Pain relief with an epidural can last throughout the entire labor and enables you to rest more, giving you more energy for pushing. It will not affect the baby and, should the need for a C-section arise, the catheter can be used to provide anesthesia. Here are the disadvantages of an epidural:

✋ You have to stay in an awkward position for about 10 minutes while the epidural is inserted, then wait another 10–20 minutes before the medication takes full effect.

✋ Depending on the type of medication you're receiving, you may not be able to stand up and move about with an epidural.

✋ Both you and the baby will require more monitoring devices.

labor and delivery

🖐 An epidural could cause your contractions to become less frequent and intense, in which case you may be given the drug Pitocin to get your labor back on track. For many women, though, the slowdown is temporary.

🖐 The loss of sensation may make it harder to push the baby out. In this case, you may choose to have the epidural dose decreased during the second stage of labor.

🖐 In rare cases, you may get patchy pain relief.

🖐 Shivering is a common reaction, although this often happens during labor even without anesthetic and will subside if you're covered with a blanket.

🖐 The drug may temporarily lower your blood pressure, slowing your baby's heart rate.

🖐 In less than 2 percent of cases, an epidural results in a bad headache. In rare instances, it can cause nerve injury or infection.

tens

TENS (or transcutaneous electrical nerve stimulation) is a method of electrical stimulation that provides you with some degree of pain relief during labor. The small, cell-phone-size machine excites sensory nerves and is connected by lead wires to electrode pads placed on particularly painful parts of your body (such as your lower back). The laboring mom can push a button for a burst of "tingles" that relieve low-level pain, and can adjust the controls to soothe chronic pain.

Apparently, TENS causes your body to release natural pain killers known as endorphins and blocks deeper pain messages from traveling to your brain. It is noninvasive and there are therefore no known side effects of this form of therapy. From what I've read (and I haven't tried it myself), TENS is most effective during early labor, but is rarely sufficient as labor contractions intensify. In fact, one study found that 8 out of 10 women who used TENS still required other methods of pain relief (drug therapy). Many women who commented on the use of TENS found that it was actually more helpful for back pain during pregnancy than during labor. But it is something that may be worth investigating, and if you do not want to use drugs during labor and are worried about your ability to bear pain, it could be worth a shot (forgive the pun).

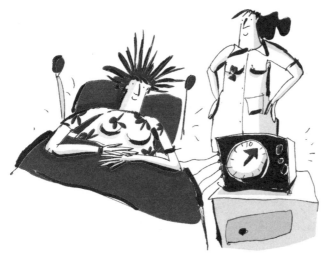

reasons for a cesarean birth

The idea of having a C-section is often terrifying to a new mom. Here are four of the most common reasons for having one, as explained by Dr. William Sears.

✋ "Failure to progress" accounts for around 30 percent of cesarean deliveries. It means that labor doesn't match the usual timetable. For various reasons, the cervix does not open enough and/or the baby does not descend. Of all the reasons for a cesarean, this is the one most under your control. Emotional and physical support, walking during labor, upright pushing, and the prudent use of medication and technology will help labor progress by increasing the efficiency of uterine contractions rather than interfering with them.

✋ A repeat cesarean (meaning that you had one previously) is the most common reason for a surgical birth, and this, too, is under your influence.

labor and delivery

Fetal distress is the third most common situation leading to a cesarean delivery. Fetal heart patterns on the electronic monitor may suggest that your baby's well-being is in jeopardy unless he or she is delivered quickly. A fetal heart rate that is higher or lower than average is a sign that your baby may not be getting enough oxygen or is not recovering well from the decreased heart rate that is normal during contractions.

Cephalopelvic disproportion (CPD) is another reason for surgical births, meaning that your baby is too big to pass through the pelvic outlet. Laboring and delivering in a more upright position (namely squatting) can enlarge the pelvic outlet, often allowing even a small mom to deliver a big baby.

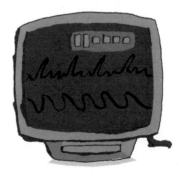

making a C-section memorable

🖐 Ask your doctor for a spinal or epidural anesthetic so that you can be awake for the birth. Have your partner sit next to you at the head of the operating table. If he's hesitant, remind him that the surgical procedure takes place behind a sterile curtain.

🖐 Ask your obstetrician to lift your baby high enough so that you can see him or her right after delivery. It is a beautiful sight to see your newborn lifted "up and out."

🖐 Immediately after your baby is delivered and checked over (for stable temperature, breathing and pulse, and heart rate) ask that he or she be brought to you to be held and hugged. You may need some help since you might be a bit groggy and one arm may be immobilized for an IV line. The anesthesiologist or pediatrician will often act as photographer.

While your uterus and abdomen are being stitched closed (this takes about 30 minutes), your partner should accompany your baby to the nursery. This extra bonding time is often recalled as having a deep effect on the partner.

To decrease post-operative pain, ask your anesthesiologist about using a long-acting analgesic called Duramorph. This do-it-yourself, "patient-controlled analgesia" (PCA) is set up so that you can administer your own medication through your IV line. Just turn the pump on and off as you need relief. This medication is safe for your breast-feeding baby.

In most cases, your baby can be brought to your bedside within an hour or two of surgery. The best post-operative "pain reliever" is an "injection" of your newborn in your arms.

breech baby?

The term "breech" refers to a baby who is not in a head-down or "vertex" position as delivery falls due; usually this means a baby who is bottom down. About 3 percent of babies at 37+ weeks' gestation are breech. Babies will usually begin turning head down between weeks 28 and 32, and continue to turn on their own, even during labor.

Some moms use nonmedical techniques to increase the chances of their baby turning into a head-down position (*see pages 406–407*). But say you've tried all of these and your baby is still breech. What does this mean? There is a lot of misinformation about the mode of birth for breech babies. Many people will tell you that the only method of delivery that is safe is an elective cesarean. This is absolutely not true: many of the problems once thought to be caused by the vaginal breech birth were actually caused by something before the birth. Less than 50 percent of all breech babies are currently being born vaginally (though this statistic varies drastically from practice to practice). As Robin Elise Weiss (a childbirth and postpartum educator, and proud mother of six) confirms, your chances of delivering a healthy breech baby vaginally increase with the following: your baby is frank breech (feet straight up); you've had a baby/babies vaginally before this birth; your baby is not thought to be excessively large; you have no pelvic or uterine anomalies.

Some breech babies are better off being born by cesarean, but only your practitioner can help you determine if your baby is one of them. This would not mean that all subsequent babies would be breech presentations or necessarily be born via cesarean section.

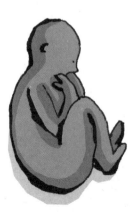

turn, baby, turn

It is worth trying the following nonmedical techniques to encourage your baby to turn head down:

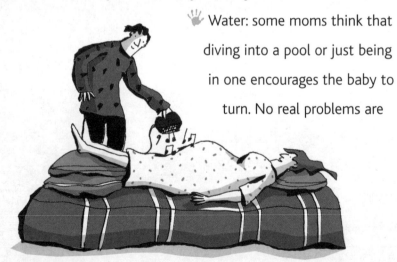 Light/music aimed directly at your pubic bone: the aim is to encourage the baby to come toward the light or sound. (A nice touch is to get your partner to talk toward your pubic bone.) Many women report success with this and it has no side effects. Do it as often as you like until your baby turns head down.

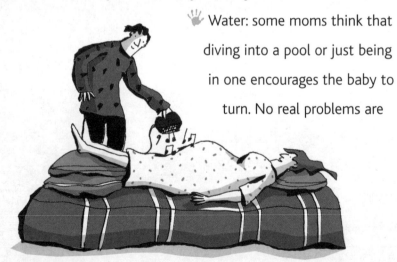 Water: some moms think that diving into a pool or just being in one encourages the baby to turn. No real problems are

noted from being in a pool, but double-check about the diving.

🖐 Tilt position: the theory is that your baby's head (the heaviest part of his or her body) will disengage from the pelvis, and your baby will turn head down. You can do this exercise using an ironing board leaning on the couch: place your feet up and your head down. Try it for 20 minutes a day until your baby turns, but discuss this or any other exercise with your midwife or doctor first.

🖐 Acupuncture: this has long been used (with moxibustion) to turn breech babies. The biggest difficulty here may be finding someone who practices these techniques.

🖐 Chiropractic care: certain chiropractic techniques may be able to help turn the baby; check with your practitioner first.

🖐 Homeopathy: remedies such as pusatilla have been used for centuries in assisting the turning of a breech baby. However, speaking to a knowledgeable practitioner is a must.

weight and blood-sugar issues

If weight or high blood sugar predispose you to having a big baby, you can take measures to minimize the possibility of having an instrumental or cesarean delivery and birth injury. These include avoiding an epidural entirely, delaying it until you are five centimeters dilated, allowing it to wear off if pushing isn't moving the baby, having no preset time limits for pushing, and pushing in an upright position. If the baby's shoulders get stuck at the birth, turning onto your hands and knees will almost always safely and effectively release them.

To prevent newborn low blood sugar, your baby should breast-feed soon after the birth, getting at least 10 minutes at each breast, especially if he or she is big, small, or the labor has been difficult. High-weight women are more likely to have high-weight children; the longer you exclusively breast-feed, the less likely your baby is to become a high-weight child.

crowning

When your baby's head is emerging through your vagina, the baby is said to be "crowning." Your midwife or doctor may ask you if you want to see the top of the baby's head in a mirror as it makes its first appearance (personally, I always told them to stick the mirror and go get the kid). Crowning is the most painful aspect of delivery, but also provides the most relief mentally, because you can see that you're almost done. Daily massage of the perineal tissues around the vaginal opening in the last six weeks of pregnancy can help reduce some of the pain of crowning and prevent the need for a nasty episiotomy (an incision in the skin between the vagina and the anus, *see pages 412–413*) to enlarge the space at the outlet.

forceps and vacuum extraction

If your baby's head keeps slipping back into the birth canal, forceps or a vacuum extractor may be used to help guide its passage. Forceps resemble two large salad spoons, and the doctor uses them to ease the baby's head out of the birth canal. Vacuum extraction involves a soft plastic cup that looks similar to an ice cream cone and is applied to the baby's head and stays in place by suction; there is a handle on the cup that allows the doctor to assist with delivery through the birth canal.

The choice between using forceps or a vacuum extractor is usually made by the doctor. These methods are sometimes used because of signs of fetal distress, prolonged second-stage labor, a difficult delivery caused by the baby's position, or the mom being too tired to push.

Studies have shown that assisting with delivery in this way does not pose any greater risk to the mother or the baby than a

C-section. When applied properly, forceps or vacuum extraction rarely causes any permanent injury to the baby: marks caused by the forceps on the baby's cheeks usually disappear in a few days, although occasionally the baby's facial nerves may be temporarily injured. The resulting drooping of facial muscles almost always recovers completely in a matter of weeks.

Caput succedaneum is diffuse swelling of the scalp caused by molding after prolonged labor, and a vacuum delivery may leave a more noticeable caput, although it usually disappears within two to three days.

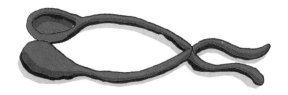

the cut

An episiotomy is an incision made in the perineum (the skin between the vagina and the anus) to avoid undue tearing as the baby passes out. It is measured in degrees—the most common being a second-degree episiotomy (midway between the vagina and the anus) and the least common a fourth-degree one (extending through the rectum). The midline is the most common form in the U.S. The American College of Obstetricians and Gynecologists says episiotomy "is not always necessary" and "should not be considered routine." However, estimates claim that the episiotomy rate in the U.S. is 65–95 percent.

An episiotomy is said to provide the following benefits: speeds up the birth; prevents tearing; protects against incontinence, protects against pelvic floor relaxation, and heals more easily than tears. These all appear to be valid reasons, but in fact medical research has not proven any of these benefits, and in many cases the opposite is actually true. The following have been reported as side effects of an episiotomy: infection, increased pain, increase in third- and fourth-degree vaginal lacerations, longer healing times, and increased discomfort when intercourse is resumed.

There is much you can do to lessen your chances of having this surgical incision. Some preventive measures include good nutrition (healthy skin stretches more easily); Kegels (exercise for your pelvic floor muscles, *see page 92*); prenatal discussion with your care provider about episiotomy; prenatal perineal massage; a slowed second stage (controlled pushing); warm compresses, perineal massage, and support during delivery. As the veteran of one very painful and unnecessary episiotomy, I can vouch for the complications and the lingering pain. So know your rights and discuss your concerns before you're in the delivery room.

post-delivery pain

After the baby arrives, you're going to feel as if you're in the middle of a hurricane. So much will be on your mind, yet your body will be telling you to sit still. Here are some ways to cope with some of the most common "ailments" after delivery. As for your need to get everything done . . . Calm down, relax, cuddle your new baby, and let everyone else help you!

You will experience a discharge of blood, called lochia, which occurs as the lining of the uterus is shed. The discharge gradually turns from a bright red to pink or brown, and finally to yellow or white before it eventually stops. It's heavy at first, but becomes lighter with time.

This bleeding will occur whether you had a vaginal delivery or a cesarean, although it's not quite as heavy with a cesarean. It should stop altogether by the time you go for your six-week postpartum checkup.

🖐 The bleeding shouldn't cause you any concern unless it suddenly becomes heavy again or you begin to pass blood clots larger than a silver dollar. In either case, call your health-care provider immediately.

🖐 You may have some pain between the vagina and the rectum. This is caused by the stretching, tearing, or cutting of the area that allowed for delivery of your baby.

🖐 If you received an episiotomy, the area where the incision was made may be quite painful, but it will heal very quickly. To ease your discomfort, you can take a shallow bath (sitz bath) that soaks your lower body and thighs.

🖐 The contractions of your uterus, which may occur for several days after the birth, signal that it is shrinking to its pre-pregnancy size. Applying warm compresses to your abdomen, or lying for a short time on a warm (not hot) heating pad, can help.

your baby's apgar score

Developed by Virginia Apgar in 1952, the Apgar score is the first test your newborn will be given right after delivery, at one minute and again at five minutes. It is given to quickly evaluate a newborn's physical condition and decide if your baby needs emergency care. If the first two scores are low, he or she will be evaluated again at 10 minutes. Five factors are used to assess your baby's condition (each factor being scored on a scale of 0–2): heart rate (pulse); breathing (rate and effort); activity and muscle tone; grimace response (known medically as "reflex irritability"); and appearance (skin coloration). These five factors are added together to calculate the Apgar score.

Although 10 is the highest possible score, babies almost never receive it because the hands and feet of healthy newborns are usually still slightly bluish at five minutes after birth (a baby has to have normal coloration all over to get the full score of 2 for appearance). A baby who scores 7 or above at one minute after birth is generally considered in good health. But a lower score doesn't necessarily mean your baby is unhealthy or abnormal (a score of 4–6 at one minute may indicate that your baby needs special immediate care, such as oxygen to help him breathe or suctioning of his airways). A newborn with an Apgar score of less than 4 generally requires advanced medical care and emergency measures, such as assisted breathing and observation in a neonatal intensive care unit (NICU). Most newborns with initial Apgar scores of less than 7 will eventually do just fine. So don't fret: worry about test scores when he's in high school!

breast-feeding

As the milk for nourishing your baby begins to flow into your breasts, they may feel sore. To ease this pain, you'll want to stimulate your breasts so that milk production can begin in earnest. The best way to do this is by encouraging your baby to breast-feed often. The more frequently (and the longer) he or she nurses, the sooner your milk production will become established.

🖐 If your breasts are painfully engorged (*see page 455*) and your baby doesn't want to feed again, you may need to apply cold compresses and to hand-express small amounts of milk often.

🖐 If you don't breast-feed, you may still feel the discomfort of engorgement. To relieve any pain, wear a supportive bra, and use an ice pack to numb the area and help dry up the milk flow.

🖐 Avoid rubbing the nipples or running warm water over the area, as both will stimulate your breasts.

🖐 If you're breast-feeding, you may be surprised at how

ravenous you feel. It's essential to have good nutrition for this important task, and your hunger ensures that you'll receive the nutrition you need. The amount of nutrients that your baby receives depends on the quality of the food you eat. Because breast-feeding places more demands on your body than pregnancy did, you need to eat an extra 500 calories a day.

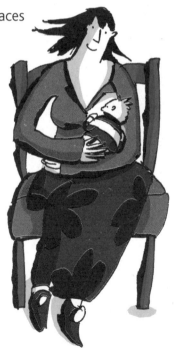 Whatever you do, don't try to diet at this point! Be good to yourself—eat foods that will provide you with the energy you need. Avoid junk food or empty-calorie foods, and drink plenty of water.

other post-delivery issues

✋ If you've had a cesarean, you'll be told to go carefully with any activity. Be cautious about lifting objects and carrying heavy items. Avoid any activities that may strain your abdominal muscles. And take care of your incision—you'll have been shown how.

✋ During this period, you might experience incontinence for a short time. If this happens, empty your bladder frequently and do your Kegel exercises. As your bladder muscles contract and grow stronger, the incontinence will pass.

✋ You may also experience uncomfortable bowel movements and hemorrhoids, and the process of delivery can also slow the movement of food through the intestines, causing you to feel bloated or constipated. Changing your diet, taking pain medication, and spending more time in bed are other factors.

✋ When you do have a bowel movement, it's important not to strain. It can help to drink plenty of fluids, to add some bran and prunes to your diet, and to take stool softeners, as recommended by your doctor.

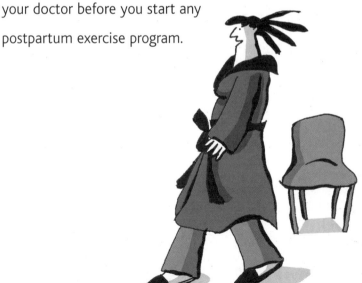 Exercise is important to your feeling of well-being after the delivery. You can begin doing very light exercises—stretching your muscles, doing Kegel exercises (*see page 92*), and walking around—while you're still in the hospital. However, check with your doctor before you start any postpartum exercise program.

new baby

I vividly remember looking down at my newborn son the morning after I had given birth and saying to him, "Hi, I'm your . . . mom." That word "mom" sounded so strange. I was someone's mother. "Wait," I thought. "Who decided that was a good idea? I can't be a mom!" But I was—and it was the best job I was ever given.

Now, if only someone had told me what to do with that stumpy-looking thing on his belly, or how to cope with my breasts that had suddenly grown into two huge, hard, hot (I mean temperature-wise) melons. Sure, my husband was impressed, but my baby thought I was insane to try to get them in his mouth. All of a sudden, I just wanted to cry—and I did, many times. But with a lot of trial and error, I managed to breast-feed, keep the umbilical stump clean (and it did fall off, eventually), and take care of my baby.

At the time of writing, my firstborn is 11 years old. Imagine that: I, who couldn't even keep a goldfish alive for a week, have managed to keep a human being alive and thriving for 11 years—and here's hoping for many more to come!

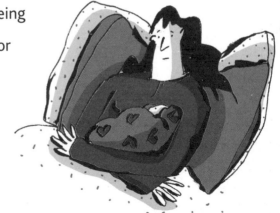

good eating habits

After the birth, you'll need all the sound nutrition you had during pregnancy—and then some. So be sure to continue your good eating habits and to take regular meals and snacks provided by your partner or other caregiver. Because many families live far away from close relatives, some new parents hire a postpartum doula, whose job it is to "mother" the mom and care for the family. But if friends offer to help, be sure to take them up on it.

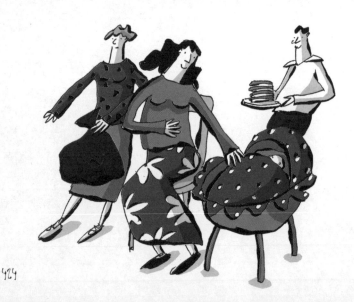

get the rest you need

You and your baby will need peace and quiet, so limit guests to friends or relatives whom you feel comfortable asking to help with the cooking and cleaning. Try to get plenty of rest for the first few days or, if you've had a cesarean, for longer. Above all, don't feel guilty about taking it easy in the first few weeks, or feel that you must do everything as soon as you get home. You need to recuperate from the hard work and physical changes of childbirth, and people will not expect you to do too much at once. Resting as much as possible will also help you to follow the advice of sleeping whenever your baby does. It is essential that you get as much sleep as possible: you took nine months to grow this baby and now you must give your body time to adjust to its nonpregnant state. Your bed is also the perfect place to cuddle your baby. A crib can be lonely, and your newborn needs the closeness of mom and dad. You'll enjoy the closeness, too!

worries about your new roles

Continuous responsibility for an infant can be an overwhelming experience for both parents. On top of this comes a major change in relationships: your twosome has suddenly become a threesome, and you're drawn compellingly into a relationship with your baby—even though you may be trying to maintain your old relationship with your partner. The birth also results in major changes for the new father. Starting with the baby's first cry, it's common for dads to feel concern about meeting the financial needs of the family. Try to take things one step at a time and not to worry about what will happen in the distant future: your whole situation may have changed by then. For now, aim to focus on the present.

new baby

unrealistic expectations

Your idea of what a "good mother" should be may have been built up to such an unrealistic level by magazine articles and books that you exhaust yourself trying to achieve it. If that happens, you may have little tolerance for the many minor problems that naturally arise during the early care of your infant. Your partner, too, may expect you quickly to start handling everything as you did before. When this doesn't occur, you may feel guilty and the father may be critical and unsympathetic. You need to settle down and just get through each day. They say practice makes perfect—well, in mothering you'll get plenty of practice, but you'll never be perfect . . . What you will become is more relaxed and less demanding of yourself. Let go of those "gold standards" of household and other work, and take each day one at a time. Don't worry if the clothes are still in the dryer— they're clean, right? What more could you ask of yourself?

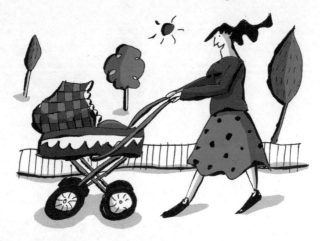

new baby

necessary losses

The joy of becoming parents is accompanied by what the writer Judith Viorst calls "necessary losses": loss of your exclusive relationship with your partner, loss of many of the activities that you participated in together, loss of daily contact with colleagues, loss of income. At this precarious time, a number of measures can help you feel less anxious. But above all, give yourself permission for rest, time out, and brief, pleasurable outings.

postpartum help

As a new mom, you need help with household chores and meal preparation for at least three to four weeks after the birth, so that you can establish a rewarding interaction with your baby and regular feedings. Today many partners arrange to take one or two weeks of vacation right after the baby's birth, and a mother, mother-in-law, or friend may also pitch in for a few days. Although such short-term support is not to be underrated, it may not give you sufficient time to become acquainted with your new baby. That's why many parents consider other sources of home help. Hiring a teenager or an older woman to help out for three hours a day, three to five days a week, can have a remarkable effect on your own life and that of your baby.

process the birth

It's helpful for all women to talk about their birth experience.
If you have good feelings about your labor and delivery,
discussing them will enhance your sense of accomplishment.
If you have negative feelings (because, for example, you felt a
lack of control or had a series of unwanted interventions), talking
about them will help you to overcome any disappointment or
sadness you may feel. You'll also begin to work through any
criticism you have about your own performance, and realize
what a remarkable feat you've achieved with the birth of your
baby. Ideally, the discussion should take place with someone
such as a nurse or doula, who was with you during labor and is
trained to be a good listener. If that's not possible, you could
write your experience down. The best time to process the birth is
after you've had a chance to rest and reflect on what happened:
two to six weeks after you return home from the hospital.

get dad to act as intermediary

The new dad will notice that if mom can sleep when the baby sleeps and not become overly tired, the postpartum period will probably proceed relatively smoothly. A particularly important role for the new father, then, is to act as a liaison with the outside world, by answering the phone and not allowing too many people to visit.

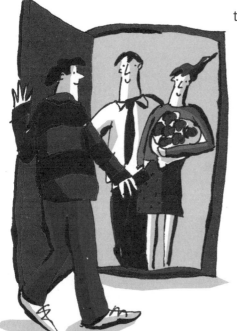

By acting as go-between in this way, dad will ensure that the new mom gets as much rest as possible.

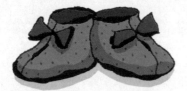

open lines of communication

For couples to bear up under the fatigue, each partner needs to make a major effort at being understanding, supportive, and communicative. It's hard to imagine just how tired you can feel when your baby's needs do not follow any normal day–night schedule. Taking turns with the nighttime watch can help, but it's equally important for both of you to express your feelings. Many moms, especially first-time ones, begin to take on the martyr complex and feel that they have to do it all. Even if dad has to get up early the next morning, you shouldn't feel bad about having him (that's right: "having him," not "asking him to") help with the baby—even at night. You'll be up early, too, and you won't be eating bonbons, so put that guilt away!

bonding with your baby

If you have time to really get to know your infant in the first few weeks, you'll feel much more confident as a mom. So use this time to keep your baby close—to hold, soothe, and love your child. When this happens, you'll find that the strong bond you develop with your baby will help you cope with the many other adjustments that you are now having to make.

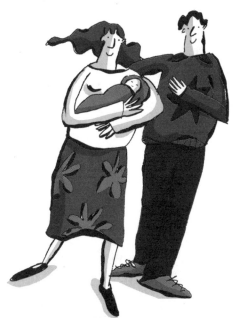

the baby blues, or ppd?

It's important to distinguish between the normal "baby blues" and true depression:

🖐 The baby blues are characterized by a short period of volatile emotions, commonly occurring between the second and fifth postpartum days and affecting 80–90 percent of new moms.

🖐 Postpartum depression (PPD) usually begins after four to eight weeks (but sometimes later in the first year) and can persist for more than a year. PPD affects 10–16 percent of new mothers. Symptoms of PPD include irritability, frequent crying, feelings of helplessness, lack of energy and motivation, disturbances of appetite and sleep, lack of interest in sex, and feelings of being unable to cope with new demands. Anxiety often shows up in lack of affection for the baby and, in turn, self-blame and guilt. PPD can have serious implications for the infant as well. A number of studies show an association between maternal depression and later developmental problems in the child, including behavioral disturbances, ill health, insecure attachments, and depression.

The outlook for moms who are suffering from PPD is good, if diagnosis and treatment are started early. When there is a significant delay, the depression may last longer. Often short-term psychotherapy is all that's needed. But the best approach is to prevent PPD in the first place, and social support is a vital factor in achieving this. Here are some suggestions: get postpartum help, seek breast-feeding support, respond to your baby's crying, set aside time for each other, and relax.

circumcision

Circumcision is a minor surgical procedure to remove the foreskin from the penis (the foreskin being a flap of skin that covers the tip of the penis at birth). Deciding whether to have your baby circumcised is often influenced by cultural, religious, and personal factors, and by the parents' assessment of the medical risks and benefits.

Generally, your baby isn't fed for an hour before circumcision. This is to prevent spitting up, since your baby will be lying on his back for the procedure.

The procedure usually takes about three to five minutes. In medical (nonritual) circumcisions, the baby is secured onto molded plastic board with Velcro straps so that he can't move much. The penis is then washed with antiseptic solution. Surgically, circumcision involves creating a thin ring of crushed tissue at the base of the foreskin where the incision is made.

new baby

The crushing of the tissue prevents bleeding. There are different sorts of instruments for protecting the tip of the penis during the procedure. Most practitioners have one technique with which they are most comfortable.

There are moments when circumcision appears to be painful, and studies have looked at newborn pain responses (such as faster heart rate and crying) and found that the procedure does cause signs of stress. Numerous techniques have been developed to provide anesthesia for circumcision.

Post-operative pain can be managed with infant acetaminophen (Tylenol), cuddling, and letting your baby suck. Some babies seem sleepy or "out of it" for a day after the procedure.

new baby

care of your baby afterward

At the end of a circumcision, the doctor will probably wrap
the tip of the penis with gauze coated in petroleum jelly
(Vaseline) to prevent any scab from sticking to the diaper.
When you change your baby's diaper, use a fresh piece of
petroleum-jellied gauze or a dab of petroleum jelly. The tip
of the penis will look red and swollen for anything from a
few days to a week afterward. A white or yellow rim may
appear where the foreskin was cut. This scab is called eschar
(pronounced "ess-car") and is part of the healing process. It will
fall off when it is ready to, and doesn't need to be pulled away.
Until fully healed (one to two weeks), the tip of your baby's
penis can be washed with plain water, dripped over from a
soaked washcloth, then patted dry. Once it looks healed, you
can discontinue using the petroleum jelly, and as long as the
umbilical cord has fallen off, start giving your baby tub baths.

new baby

introducing an older child

When a new baby is first brought home, Dr. Benjamin Spock says, "It may be better for the older child to be away on an excursion, if this can be arranged. An hour later, when the baby and the luggage are in their place and the mother is at last relaxing on the bed, is time enough for the child to come in. His mom can hug him and talk to him and give him her undivided attention. Since children appreciate concrete rewards, it's nice to bring a present home for the sibling." It's probably best not to keep asking the older child if he likes his new sister or brother.

the umbilical cord

When still in the mother's womb, the baby is nourished through the blood vessels of the umbilical cord. Just after birth, the doctor puts a plastic clamp on the cord and cuts it off close to the baby's body. A stump is left, and this withers like a raisin and eventually drops off—usually in about two or three weeks, though it may take a little longer.

If the cord hasn't fallen off one month after the birth, mention this to your child's doctor, although most doctors and nurses don't become concerned until it has hung on for six weeks or longer.

To help the cord dry out, fold down the top of your baby's

new baby

diaper so that the cord is exposed to the air. To keep it dry, give your baby sponge baths (rather than regular baby baths), using a damp, soft cloth to wipe off your baby's head, body, arms, and legs. It's best to give only sponge baths until the cord has fallen off and the navel has scabbed over (usually at two to six weeks).

If a little water drips on the cord during a sponge bath, just use a soft cloth to dry it off afterward. Many parents use a cotton swab dipped in rubbing alcohol to gently wash around the base of the cord. You can also use premoistened, individually wrapped alcohol swabs. The alcohol keeps the area clean and helps the cord to dry out.

You can pick up the cord with one hand and gently move it left, right, up, and down, so that you clean around it. The cord has no nerve endings and so cannot feel pain. But if you rub too vigorously on the skin around the cord, it will become irritated.

when the cord falls off

After the cord falls off, it leaves a raw spot, which takes a number of days (or occasionally a few weeks) to heal. The raw spot should merely be kept clean and dry so that it won't get infected. If it is kept dry, a scab will cover it until it is healed. It doesn't need a bandage and will stay drier without one.

Once the cord falls off, your baby can have tub baths. Just dry the navel afterward with a corner of the towel (or absorbent cotton balls, if you like) until it is all healed.

There may be a bit of bleeding or seeping of clear fluid a few days before the cord falls off and until the healing is complete (or if clothing pulls off the scab). If there is more blood, or if oozing persists for more than a few hours, talk to your doctor.

Continue to keep the diaper below the level of the unhealed navel so that it stays dry. If the navel produces a moist discharge, clean it each day with a cotton swab dampened with alcohol.

If the skin around the navel becomes red or tender, or there is a smelly discharge, it may be a sign of infection, so contact your health-care provider right away. It's normal to note a little odor just as the cord is coming off, particularly when it becomes soft.

If healing is slow and the navel continues to be moist, the raw spot may become lumpy with "granulation tissue." This is nothing to worry about—the doctor may apply silver nitrate to hasten healing and make the lumpiness go away. In rare cases, you might notice yellowish fluid or even a bit of bowel movement leaking out—this is treatable, so just be sure to tell your doctor.

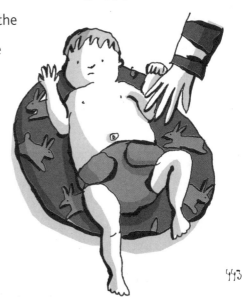

blocked tear ducts

Normally, tears are cleared from the eye through small tubes known as tear ducts that extend from the eye into the nose. When these ducts are blocked, a baby's tears flow down his or her cheek or build up and dry out, leaving clumps of yellowish discharge or matter in the eye.

Blocked tear ducts are very common in newborns and young babies. Although they can be a nuisance, they almost never pose a serious problem. The buildup of discharge makes a baby more prone to eye infections, so until the ducts open, be sure to clean your infant's eyes very gently with a piece of absorbent cotton dipped in cooled boiled water; sometimes a warm compress helps loosen the secretions and makes them easier to remove. Ask your health-care provider to show you how best to clean your child's eyes.

Blocked tear ducts generally open up by themselves within the first few weeks or months of life. Sometimes massaging the ducts helps them open sooner, so ask your care provider if massaging the ducts will help in your child's case.

🖐 Once in a while, a minor surgical procedure is required to open them up. Your practitioner will let you know if the time comes to explore this kind of treatment.

🖐 If the amount of discharge increases, or if the white part of your child's eyelids becomes red or swollen, he or she may have developed an infection, even if there isn't a telltale fever. If your child develops these symptoms, he or she should be checked by your health-care provider so that a course of antibiotics can be prescribed, if necessary.

thrush

Thrush is a yeast (candida) infection of the mouth that is most commonly seen in otherwise healthy infants. According to Lynn Cates, M.D., it looks like white patches of milk, or "cheesy" material, on the inside of the cheeks, gums, palate, and tongue. You can tell that it isn't milk because it won't rinse off, and if you try to scrape it off, you may see some bleeding.

Most babies aren't bothered at all by mild thrush, but some have sufficient pain to make them fussy and interfere with their ability to suck and swallow normally. Most of the time, thrush can be diagnosed just by looking at the rash.

Mild cases may go away without treatment, but others might need an over-the-counter remedy or a prescription for a liquid medicine called nystatin. Unlike most other medicines, you don't want your baby to swallow this one right away because it needs to have contact with the rash to kill the yeast. So be sure to put it into the front of your child's mouth, and don't give her anything to eat or drink for at least a half hour afterward. You may find it easier to get it into the right part of the mouth by using your finger to "paint" the medicine right onto the thrush.

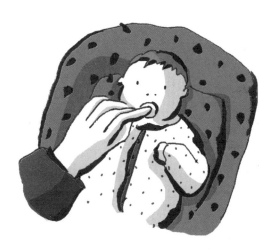 Thrush can cause rashes literally at both ends. So if your baby has diaper rash at the same time as thrush, she may need nystatin cream or ointment for her diaper area.

preventing reinfection

It is important to prevent thrush reinfection by getting rid of yeast from surfaces that come into contact with your infant's mouth. These include treating candida skin infections on the breast, if a baby is breast-feeding; and washing bottles, nipples, and pacifiers with hot, soapy water, then boiling them to eliminate yeast. If the thrush persists, consider buying new bottles and a new pacifier.

If you have sharp, shooting pains in your breasts, or your nipples become red and shiny, it is essential that your nipples and your baby's mouth be treated for thrush, even if there is no obvious sign of the infection.

baby pimples

Baby acne is thought to occur in part because of exposure to the mom's hormones during pregnancy. Unfortunately, the condition commonly lasts for several months and there's really nothing you can do to treat it. Simply use water to clean your baby's skin, and don't apply any lotion or baby oil, which can exacerbate the acne. And don't pick the pimples—this only makes them worse!

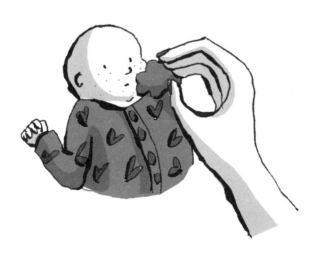

pacifiers

A baby who has periods of mild irritability can often be entirely quieted by having a pacifier to suck. Dr. Benjamin Spock says, "We don't know whether this is true because the sucking soothes some vague discomfort or whether it simply keeps the baby occupied with a deep-seated reflex to suck."

Pacifiers are helpful for babies who are sucking down bottle after bottle of formula—sometimes as much as 40 oz (1.1 kg) per day. Often what these babies really need is more time sucking, and a pacifier can give them this, without the unneeded calories.

The pacifier, when used correctly, can also prevent thumb-sucking. Most babies who freely use a pacifier for the first months of life never become thumb-suckers, even if they give up the pacifier at three to four months.

The best time to offer a pacifier is whenever the baby is searching around with his or her mouth and trying to suck on anything that is handy. The idea is to give the pacifier to your child as much as he can use it in the first three months, so that he will be satisfied and able to readily give it up later on.

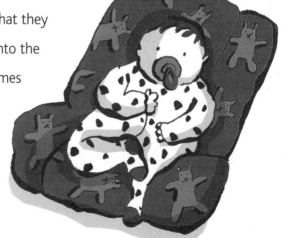 Two problems can interfere with efficient use of the pacifier. In some cases, parents are reluctant to use it at all, or try it so late that the baby won't take to it. In other cases, they may have developed such a dependence on it—for comforting the baby when she so much as whimpers—that they can't stop popping it into the baby's mouth many times a day, even after she is ready to give it up (usually at two to four months).

pacifiers in bed

If your baby is still on a pacifier after five or six months and is waking several times a night because he's lost it, put several in the bed at bedtime so that there's a better chance of his finding one by himself. Or let it stay lost; this could be a good time to get him used to doing without it.

Never put a long cord on a pacifier to hang it around your baby's neck or tie it to the crib bar. This can be dangerous, because the cord might become wrapped around the baby's finger, wrist, or neck, and might cause injury or even death.

🖐 Replace old pacifiers before they become too worn. When a baby has a few teeth, he can pull the nipple of an old, tired pacifier off the disk or chew pieces out of the nipple. These broken-off pieces may cause serious choking if they are swallowed the wrong way. So buy new pacifiers before the old ones become at all weak or crumbly.

🖐 Clean pacifiers frequently with warm, soapy water. Pacifiers can become contaminated with candida, the yeastlike fungi that causes thrush (*see pages 446–447*). If your baby develops thrush, you'll need to sterilize the pacifier by placing it in boiling water for 10 minutes to get rid of any remaining sources of infection.

cradle cap

What is this scaly stuff on your perfect child's head? I always called it baby dandruff, but its proper name is cradle cap. It is fairly common and normally goes away on its own, usually within weeks. However, more severe cases may affect other parts of the body (usually the face), causing itchiness. Generally, washing with mild soap and water will eliminate cradle cap, but if it seems to be drying out, try a little olive oil.

After a couple of treatments with olive oil, both of my boys were free of it. If it spreads, talk to your pediatrician about medications or shampoos.

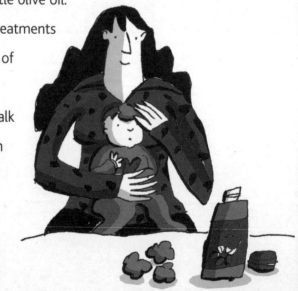

engorgement

Engorgement is defined as swollen, hard breasts, but if your baby feeds frequently, engorgement will probably be relieved within 48 hours. To keep the areola soft so that your baby can latch on to feed, try the following:

🖐 Apply moist heat to the breast before feeding, expressing enough colostrum or milk to soften the areola.

🖐 Stand in a hot shower with the water at your back, letting it run over your shoulders and breasts. Express or pump milk while in the shower.

🖐 You might need to limit the time that your baby feeds on the first breast, to make sure he or she will take the second breast during the feeding.

🖐 Cold packs (or frozen veggies!) might relieve pain and swelling, if used after feeding.

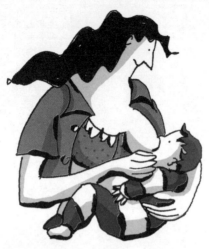

establishing a good milk supply

The amount of milk you produce is directly related to the amount of stimulation your breasts receive. Breast-feeding time should not be limited, and ideally both breasts should be used at each feeding (alternating the starting sides), but ensure the first breast is emptied before starting on the second. If your baby has trouble latching on by day three, call a lactation consultant. Remember that nursing moms need plenty of fluids—if you drink something every time you nurse your baby, you will stay hydrated, but avoid caffeine and alcohol, which encourage fluid loss; your urine should be pale in color. Breast-feeding is enhanced if you are comfortable and relaxed at feedings. And having your baby positioned properly at the breast is important in avoiding sore nipples and ensuring an adequate supply. Be sure to

✋ find a comfortable position, sitting up or lying down. Your baby's tummy should be facing your tummy.

✋ support your breast with your hand, with your thumb on top and your fingers underneath.

✋ stimulate your baby to arouse interest, tickling his or her lips to open the mouth, then quickly bring your baby to your breast.

✋ be patient and keep trying—this is a learned skill.

✋ at every feeding, get the nipple and a good portion of the areola well back into the baby's mouth.

sore nipples

Sore nipples usually result from improper positioning. If you feel sore, review your position and follow these steps:

- Your baby should feed first on the less sore side.

- Short, frequent feedings are better than long, infrequent ones.

- Change your feeding position so that your baby's jaws exert pressure on less sore areas.

- Remember to remove your baby from the breast by breaking the suction with your finger.

- After each feeding, wipe your baby's saliva from the nipple, express a few drops of breast milk on the nipple area to promote healing, and air-dry your breasts for 15–20 minutes.

positive signs

Signs that breast-feeding is going well include the following:

🖐 Your baby is feeding well 8–12 times every 24 hours.

🖐 His or her urine is pale in color.

🖐 Your baby wets at least six diapers every 24 hours after the third day. (If your baby is not having at least six wet diapers every 24 hours by day five, call your pediatrician.)

🖐 Bowel movements are soft and mustard colored by the end of the first week; they may be frequent, and the amount will vary.

🖐 Your baby regains birth weight by two to three weeks of age and continues to gain at a steady rate.

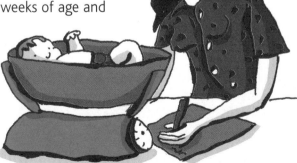

can't breast-feed?

Even though I breast-fed all of my children, I have babysat often enough to know that bottle feeding works just fine! If you can't breast-feed—or don't want to—here are some tips to start you off:

🖐 Most babies enjoy their formula slightly warmed, so run warm tap water over the bottle for several minutes, then shake a few drops on your inner wrist to check the temperature.

🖐 To minimize air swallowing, tilt the bottle, allowing the milk to fill the nipple and the air to rise to the bottom of the bottle.

🖐 Keep your baby's head straight in relation to the rest of the body. Drinking while the head is turned sideways or tilted back makes it more difficult for him or her to swallow.

🖐 To lessen arm fatigue and present different views to your baby, switch arms at each feeding.

🖐 Watch for signs that the nipple hole is too large or too small. If your baby gets a sudden mouthful of milk and sputters and

almost chokes during a feed, the milk flow may be too fast.
Turn the full bottle upside down without shaking it; if milk flows
instead of drips, the nipple hole is too large, so discard the nipple.
If your baby seems to be working hard, tires easily during sucking,
and his cheeks cave in because of a strong vacuum, the hole may
be too small (formula should drip at least one drop per second).

Know when to quit: babies know when they've had enough.
If your baby falls into a deep sleep near the end of
the feeding, but has not finished the bottle, stop.
Often babies fall into a light sleep toward the
end, but continue a flutter
type of sucking. Remove
the bottle and let them
suck for a few minutes
on your fingertip.

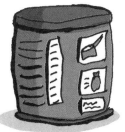

cloth diapers: the pros

Reusable and made of soft cotton, these are the old-fashioned kind of diapers that your grandmother (and maybe even your mother) used. They come either prefolded (with a center strip more absorbent than the outer strips) or flat (so that you can fold them to the shape you want), and must be used with some kind of waterproof cover to keep your baby's clothes dry. (Several brands combine a cotton diaper with a built-in cover.)

Advocates of cotton diapers say they are more comfortable (i.e., softer), more healthful (because they're free of chemicals), and more environmentally friendly than disposables, because they're reusable and won't end up clogging landfill sites.

🖐 In some ways, they are also more convenient: if you use a diaper service, they'll bring you a nice pile of fresh, snowy-white diapers every week, and you don't have to haul those bulky packages of disposables home from the store.

🖐 Cloth diapers can also save you money. Disposable diapers can set you back between $36 and $100 a month (depending on the age of your baby), so over three years you might shell out $2,000 for diapers alone. But buying, say, four dozen diapers for your growing child (at about $25 per dozen), plus a range of diaper covers, and then washing them yourself, can cost you as little as $300 over three years. Of course, diaper services can cost up to $60 a month, so over three years you might spend some $2,000 on this service, plus another $100 on wraps or covers.

cloth diapers: the cons

Before you pat yourself on the back for saving the earth (and your family some bucks) by going with cloth, you should realize that the argument is not that straightforward.

✋ For one thing, the environmental claim is debatable. Cotton diapers require both energy and water to wash them, which can make them an ecological liability, especially in regions that are short of those resources. Most cotton also requires heavy amounts of pesticides to grow, and diaper services may use harsh chemicals or chlorine for washing. And diaper-service trucks use gas to deliver their wares and disgorge pollutants into the air as they tootle around town. You can buy organic cotton diapers to solve the pesticide problem, but they're more expensive. If you forgo the diaper service, washing your own diapers in environmentally friendly detergents and drying them on a clothesline will reduce their ecological cost.

✳ Cloth diapers also entail extra work: If you have a diaper service, you must put out your dirty diapers for collection every week, and you'll probably need to fold them before you put them away. If you reuse your own cotton diapers, you'll need to wash them. This isn't as bad as it sounds—just shake out any fecal matter into the toilet, soak the dirty diapers in a pail of water with vinegar or baking soda, then throw them in the wash.

✳ As far as your baby's comfort is concerned, you must be scrupulous about changing cloth diapers when they get wet, or he or she can end up with diaper rash (*see pages 470–471*).

✳ And unless you wrap very carefully, cotton diapers can leak more than disposables do.

✳ Finally, many day-care centers won't use cotton diapers (because of convenience and hygiene concerns), so you might end up buying disposables for the center even if you use cloth ones at home.

disposables: pros and cons

Just as cloth has its pros and cons, so do disposables. So, what's a parent to do? Try them both, and see which you like best. I liked cloth more and more as my baby turned into a toddler, because it made potty training 10 times easier. And I hated that gel stuff that comes out of disposables during a particularly wet night. Cloth also always gave me something soft to put next to a rash.

The advantage of disposables is that they are easy to put on and remove, readily available, and preferred by day-care centers. They hold much more urine and can fit more snugly than cloth diapers, preventing leakage.

And many people say that disposables are better at warding off diaper rash, because they absorb urine quickly and lock it in layers, away from the baby's skin. Best of all, you won't face stacks of urine- and feces-soiled diapers on laundry day.

There are also downsides. First, they are more expensive (*see page 463*). Second, they fill up landfills with plastic material that is slow to decompose and with baby feces that pollutes the ground water. Third, a recent German study (published in the *British Medical Journal*, May 2000) has suggested a possible link between disposables and both testicular cancer and low sperm counts when boy babies grow up; more research is needed, but the study gave many parents pause for thought. Fourth, many parents don't change disposables as often as they should, as they think their baby is being kept dry. Finally, dirty diapers in your garbage can smell really bad unless they're wrapped in even more plastic.

diapering accessories

You didn't think you needed just diapers, did you? Here are a few other accessories you might want to have on hand.

🖐 Diaper bags now come in a variety of styles and sizes, from backpacks to duffel bags. Many feature pull-out or detachable changing pads with easy-to-clean surfaces, adjustable straps, roomy storage pockets, and bottle holders. Partly as a nod to all the baby-toting modern dads out there, the cutesy prints that were *de rigueur* seem to have been upstaged by unisex colors such as black, navy, and red. There's even a sleek black model that is almost indistinguishable from a briefcase. Depending on the features, they range from around $15 to more than $100.

🖐 Diaper wipes are moist towelettes specially designed for wiping urine and feces off your baby's bottom. For a newborn, look for a type that's free of perfume and alcohol, both of which can irritate your baby's sensitive skin. (Or use warm water on a

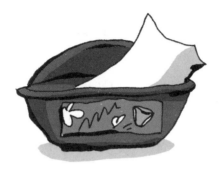

soft washcloth, or heavy tissues.) An older baby can usually tolerate wipes with a fragrance; just be sure to discontinue their use if a rash, scaling, or any other sign of irritation appears on your baby's bottom. Remember: you don't have to use a wipe if your baby only peed, and no matter what came out of her body, wipe gently on that sensitive skin.

A wipe warmer isn't exactly a "necessity," but there's something rather comforting about the thought of using one, especially on cold winter nights. Just plug the unit in (most use very little electricity), pop in your wipes, and they will be gently warmed up to a soothing temperature. Most models cost around $20.

diarrhea and diaper rash

Irritating bowel movements during an attack of diarrhea sometimes cause a very sore rash around the anus or a smooth, bright red rash on the buttocks. The treatment is to try to change the diaper just as soon as it is soiled—no small task. Clean the irritated or raw areas with warm water, gently pat the area dry, and apply a thick covering of diaper cream or an ointment made from petroleum jelly and lanolin. If this doesn't work, the diaper should be left off and the diaper area exposed to the air. Sometimes it seems that while the baby has diarrhea, nothing helps very much. Fortunately, this type of diaper rash normally cures itself as soon as the diarrhea is over. However, if your baby's rash persists or continues to worsen despite your efforts, beyond the time when the diarrhea resolves, or if your baby seems to be in considerable pain, get the rash evaluated by your child's health-care provider. It's a good idea always to have plenty of extra diaper wipes on hand, to save your household from the horrors of running out when your eight-month-old suddenly develops diarrhea in the middle of the night. If you stock up on wipes, only to find that your child is potty trained sooner than you expected, they come in handy for sticky fingers and faces long after the diaper days are over.

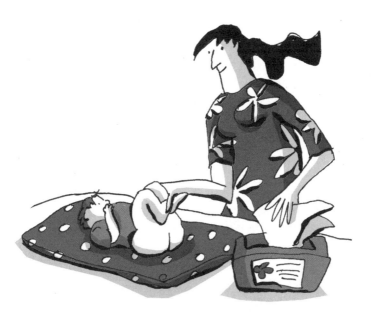

glossary

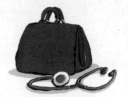

Alpha fetoprotein (AFP)
An antigen present in the fetus.
AFP blood tests are done at
15–17 weeks of pregnancy to
detect neural-tube defects and
Down's syndrome.

Amniocentesis A test that
takes a sample of amniotic
fluid to determine whether
the baby has a chromosomal
disorder or fetal lung
immaturity. It is done from
15 weeks of pregnancy.

Apgar score A test to evaluate
the newborn's status during
the first five minutes of life.
Apgar is scored on heartrate,
breathing, muscle tone, reflex
irritability, and color, each
having a value of 0 to 2.

Braxton Hicks contraction
A fake, intermittent, painless
uterine contraction that may
occur every 10–20 minutes,
any time after the third month
of pregnancy. Named after
John Braxton Hicks (1823–97),
a British gynecologist who first
described them in 1872.

Breech A variation of the
normal head-down (vertex)
presentation of the baby,
in which the buttocks are
presenting first.

Cervical dilation The
stretching and opening of
the entrance to the uterus.

Cervix The neck of the uterus.

Cesarean section (C-section)
Surgical delivery of the baby
through an incision made in
the mother's abdominal wall
and uterus.

**Chorionic villus sampling
(CVS)** A test to detect
chromosomal abnormalities in
the baby, by removal of tissue
from fingerlike projections
known as villi in the baby's
placenta. It is done from 10
weeks of pregnancy.

CNM Certified Nurse Midwife.

Crowning The point during
labor at which the baby's head
emerges through the vagina.

Doula An experienced labor
companion who provides
continuous emotional support
and assistance before, during,
and after the birth.

Edema A local or generalized
condition in which the body
tissues retain an excessive
amount of fluid.

Effacement The shortening, or
thinning, of the cervical canal as
the cervix dilates.

**Electronic fetal monitoring
(EFM)** A monitoring procedure,
either internal or external, used
to detect complications in labor.

Engagement The point at
which the widest diameter of
the baby's presenting part has
passed through the pelvic inlet.

Epidural A regional anesthetic
given at the base of the spine
(the epidural space) to stop
messages of pain from being
sent to the brain, thus partially
or completely eliminating the
sensation of pain in childbirth.

Episiotomy An incision made in the perineum at the end of the second stage of labor to avoid tearing and ease delivery.

Fetal lie The position of the baby *in utero*, also known as presentation.

Hypertension A blood pressure reading of 140/90 or higher on at least two occasions, six hours apart.

Hypoxia Lack of oxygen to the baby.

Induction The starting of labor by artificial means.

IV line Intravenous line.

Kegel exercise An exercise to contract and release the muscles of the pelvic floor to help prepare for labor.

Mucous plug The plug of mucus that seals the entrance to the cervix. When it falls out, a "bloody show" results and is a sign the baby is on the way.

Oral glucose tolerance testing (OGTT) A blood test to screen for gestational diabetes or glucose intolerance. It is done from 28 weeks of pregnancy.

Patient-controlled analgesia (PCA) Medication that is set up so that the mother can administer her own medication through an IV line.

Perineum The skin between the vagina and the anus.

Pitocin A drug used to induce or augment labor by causing potent and selective stimulation of the uterine and mammary gland muscles.

Placenta A temporary organ, which anchors the developing fetus to the uterus and creates a bridge for the exchange of nutrients, oxygen, protective antibodies, and waste products.

Placenta previa When the placenta lies over the cervix; it usually leads to a C-section.

Pre-eclampsia The development of hypertension, protein in the urine, swelling, and/or changes in certain blood tests. Also known as toxemia or pregnancy-induced hypertension.

Rhesus (Rh factor) An antigen in the blood that some people (known as Rh-positive) have and others (Rh-negative) don't. It can cross the placenta and attack the fetus' red blood cells, but is preventable with Rh-immunoglobulin medication.

Transcutaneous electrical nerve stimulation (TENS) A method of electrical stimulation that provides some degree of pain relief during labor.

Ultrasound The transmission of high-frequency soundwaves to outline various tissues in the womb. Ultrasound testing is done from about 18 weeks, with a vaginal or abdominal probe, to evaluate the pregnancy.

VBAC Vaginal Birth After Cesarean.

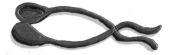

resources

Useful web sites

www.babycenter.com
www.childbirth.org
www.cpsc.gov
www.dona.org
www.epregnancy.com
www.fitpregnancy.com
www.morningsicknesshelp.com
www.morningwell.com
www.mothering.com
www.onlineclothingstores.com/Maternity.htm
www.naturalchildbirth.org
www.parentsplace.com
www.pregnancytoday.com
www.thelaboroflove.com
www.toejam.net

Useful organizations

The Bradley Method
Promotes the Bradley method
of natural childbirth.

American Academy of
Husband-Coached Childbirth
Box 5224
Sherman Oaks
CA 91413-5224
Tel: 800-4-A-BIRTH
www.bradleybirth.com

La Leche League
Promotes a better understanding of
breastfeeding; a great pregnancy resource
and helpful after the birth too.

Tel: 1-800-LALECHE (US) or 847-519-7730
www.lalecheleague.org

**International Childbirth Education
Association (ICEA), Inc.**
Unites those who believe in freedom of choice
based on knowledge of the alternatives in
family-centered maternity and newborn care.

PO Box 20048
Minneapolis
MN 55420
Tel: 952-854-8660
www.icea.org

**International Cesarean Awareness
Network (ICAN), Inc.**
Non-profit organization founded to improve
maternal–child health by preventing
unnecessary cesareans, providing support for
cesarean recovery, and promoting VBAC.

1304 Kingsdale Avenue
Redondo Beach
CA 90278
Tel: 800-686-ICAN or 310-542-6400
www.ican-online.org

Further reading

James F. Clapp III, *Exercising Through Your Pregnancy*, Addicus Books, 2002

Ginny Graves and *Fitness* magazine, *Pregnancy Fitness: Mind, Body, Spirit*, Three Rivers Press, 1999

A. Christine Harris, *The Pregnancy Journal: A Day-To-Day Guide to a Healthy and Happy Pregnancy*, Chronicle Books, 1996

Vicki Iovine, *The Girlfriends' Guide to Pregnancy*, Pocket Books, 1995

Sheila Kitzinger, *The Complete Book of Pregnancy and Childbirth*, Knopf, 4th edition 2003

Heidi E. Murkoff, Arlene Eisenberg, Sandee Hathaway, *What to Expect When You're Expecting*, Workman Publishing Company, 3rd edition 2002

William and Martha Sears, *The Birth Book: Everything You Need to Know to Have a Safe and Satisfying Birth*, Little Brown, 1994

William and Martha Sears, *The Breast Feeding Book: Everything You Need to Know About Nursing Your Child . . .* , Little Brown, 2000

Martha Rose Shulman and Jane M. D. Davis, *Every Woman's Guide to Eating During Pregnancy*, Houghton Mifflin, 2002

Elizabeth Somer, *Nutrition for a Healthy Pregnancy: The Complete Guide to Eating Before, During, and After Your Pregnancy*, Henry Holt, 1995

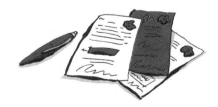

index

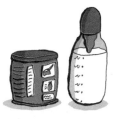

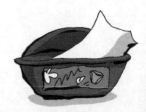

acknowledgments

First and foremost, I would like to thank my children—Matt, Lydia, Alex, and Liam—for four of the most enjoyable pregnancies and natural childbirths a mother could have. I would also like to thank my husband, John Hogan, for supporting me always and for chiming in a tip here and there when I was stuck.

To all of the mothers and fathers who contributed tips and ideas, I am very grateful for your willingness to share your experiences. And to Rebecca Saraceno, Mandy Greenfield, Sophie Collins, and Patty Moosbrugger, who made writing this book both an enjoyable and educational experience.

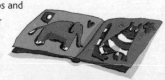